Your
Natural
BABY

Your *Natural* BABY

Complementary Therapies for the First Three Years

ANNE CHARLISH

Consultant
Dr Leo Stimmler MD FRCP

Photography by
Laura Wickenden

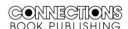

CONNECTIONS
BOOK PUBLISHING

To Gill and Dot with warmest thanks.

ADVICE TO THE READER
This book is not intended as guidance for the treatment of serious health problems;
please refer to a medical professional if you are in any doubt about
any aspect of an infant's condition.

A CONNECTIONS BOOK

This edition published in Great Britain in 1996 by
Connections Book Publishing Limited
St Chad's House
148 King's Cross Road
London WC1X 9DH

1 3 5 7 9 10 8 6 4 2

British Library Cataloguing in Publication data

Charlish, Anne
Your natural baby: complementary therapies for the first
three years
1. Infants – Care 2. Naturopathy 3. Infants – Development
I. Title
649.1'22

ISBN 1-85906-005-6

Phototypeset in Baskerville No. 2 and Americana Bold
using QuarkXpress on Apple Macintosh.
Origination by Sele & Color, Italy.
Printed and bound in Singapore by Star Standard Industries PTE Ltd.

Contents

Foreword

Throughout the last century or so, medical scientists have attempted to evaluate remedies scientifically. This has been easy for some conditions; there is however a host of diseases as yet without an obvious remedy. Provided the illness can be carefully defined, one can calculate the effectiveness of any particular therapy. If a treatment group of patients does significantly better than a control group, then one can say the therapy is of help.

But this cannot apply if the symptoms presented by a patient, whether adult or child, are not part of a well-defined disease entity. I would say that on average seven out of ten out-patients I see fall into this category. Orthodox medicine treats many and often serious conditions. But it is unable to relieve a vast range of symptoms and/or diseases that can be neither diagnosed nor analysed. To many sufferers it is the wide range of complementary therapies that offers an alternative. Though they cannot be scientifically evaluated, for many people – particularly when engendering good health in babies and their parents – such therapies have proved to be of significant help.

Dr Leo Stimmler, Consultant Paediatrician, Guy's Hospital, London, England, 1996

Introduction

This is the first book to focus in such depth on bringing up your child throughout her first three years with the benefit of a broad range of complementary theories. It is a fitting successor to *Your Natural Pregnancy*.

Nearly half of all British family doctors now refer patients for some form of complementary therapy, according to research published in 1995 by the Department of Health. In 1993, after many years of scepticism, the British Medical Association accepted that such therapies have an important part to play in the relief of a number of conditions and illnesses.

It is important to note that the therapies featured in this book are correctly termed 'complementary'. They are not presented as alternative therapies to orthodox medicine. Conventional medicine and orthodox hospital treatment have their place, and it is for this reason that the A–Z of conditions and illnesses, the substance of Part Three, is deliberately designed not to encourage home diagnosis. Once you have the diagnosis, it is safe to proceed to treatment as shown in the book.

How the Therapies Work

It is true that each therapy works in a highly complex and individualistic way. However, the therapies share a number of features. Each is intended to treat and benefit the whole adult or child rather than merely the symptoms. Each therapy is designed to stimulate the body's immune system and marshall the body's defences in order to fight against ill health. Disturbances in the pattern of the body's energies and life forces can be resolved by one or other of the therapies featured in the first part of the book.

Osteopathy, for example, aims to integrate the whole child so that all the body's systems will function more effectively and therefore be able to deal with any disease conditions that arise. In this way almost any condition, from allergies and anxiety to asthma and infectious diseases, can be treated by integrating the structure of the body in order to improve its function. Kinesiology is another therapy that seeks to identify and correct disturbances in the patterns and flow of the body's energy.

Because the complementary therapies seek to stimulate the body's defences in order to fight ill health, the condition can often worsen before it starts to get better. Homoeopathy is a good example of this feature. Treating like with like, as homoeopathy does, means that the body is subjected, for the moment, to more of what caused the illness in the first place; this boosts the body's natural defences and promotes swift healing.

Choosing a Therapy

There is no reason why you should elect one particular therapy to the exclusion of all the others to boost your child's health. It is perfectly possible to use one therapy for one ailment, a second for a different disease, and a third for another problem. What is important, however, is that each practitioner you consult is aware of what other therapies you and your child are using. There can, for example, sometimes be conflicts between aromatherapy, herbalism and homoeopathy.

Many of you will already be familiar with the mainstream complementary therapies and be happy to use them to treat your child. May I suggest that you now consider the less well-known therapies, such as kinesiology, cranio-sacral therapy, sound therapy and colour therapy; these too will become part of the mainstream in time. Colour, for example, has a profound influence on our perception, thought processes and emotions, but it may take some

years for this to be fully recognized. The Useful Addresses section (*see page 157*) gives details of how to locate a practitioner of your chosen therapy in your area.

How the Book Works

Part One aims to describe the principles and practice of the selected therapies. How to use the therapy at home is also covered. The therapies include naturopathy, massage, aromatherapy, herbalism, Bach flower remedies, homoeopathy, colour therapy, Bates eyesight training, kinesiology, the Alexander technique, osteopathy and chiropractic, cranio-sacral therapy, and movement and dance.

Part Two shows you how you may put the therapies into practice at home day by day and week by week. This part of the book is concerned, within its chronological framework, with realizing your child's potential in physical, creative, emotional and social terms and with resolving troublesome ailments, many of which are seen as commonplaces of childhood.

The third part of the book focuses on the conditions and illnesses that may beset any child up to the age of three years, showing primarily how such afflictions can be treated by one or more of the complementary therapies. As noted earlier in this Introduction, Part Three is not designed to be a home diagnosis manual. Whenever you are in any doubt whatsoever about the well-being of your child, do not hesitate to seek professional help.

Finally, I wish to thank the team of specialist practitioners for their valuable contributions. I hope that as the successor to *Your Natural Pregnancy* this book will help you to realize your child's full potential as well as making your parenting years a fully rewarding and happy period of your life.

Anne Charlish, Sussex, England, 1996

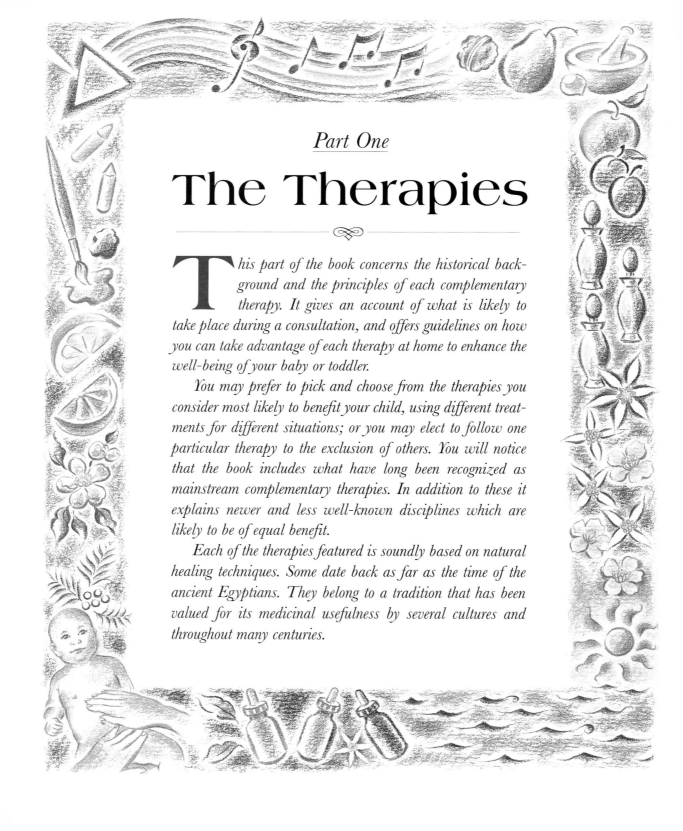

Part One

The Therapies

❧

This part of the book concerns the historical background and the principles of each complementary therapy. It gives an account of what is likely to take place during a consultation, and offers guidelines on how you can take advantage of each therapy at home to enhance the well-being of your baby or toddler.

You may prefer to pick and choose from the therapies you consider most likely to benefit your child, using different treatments for different situations; or you may elect to follow one particular therapy to the exclusion of others. You will notice that the book includes what have long been recognized as mainstream complementary therapies. In addition to these it explains newer and less well-known disciplines which are likely to be of equal benefit.

Each of the therapies featured is soundly based on natural healing techniques. Some date back as far as the time of the ancient Egyptians. They belong to a tradition that has been valued for its medicinal usefulness by several cultures and throughout many centuries.

Naturopathy

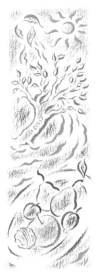

The birth of a baby and its early years of growth and development are a remarkable fulfilment of nature's intentions. Complex changes within our bodies are taking place from our earliest moments as human beings guided by an inherent vitality which we all possess. Naturopathy is a system of medicine which recognizes this vitality and applies the wisdom of nature in a scientific way to encourage and enable our own self-healing processes to work. The tools to assist this are often simple and readily available in your own home – basic natural foods, gentle massage, water treatments, fresh air, and so on. Such means ensure that naturopathy is an ideal system of healthcare for babies and young children.

Its guiding principle – only nature heals – emphasizes the remarkable abilities of our own bodies to recover from many acute and chronic ailments given the right resources. This is especially so for babies and young children, and nurturing them according to naturopathic principles will help you to give them the best possible start in life.

Naturopaths advocate a lifestyle which shows respect for nature and its expression in the growth and development of the young person. Of course, working more closely with nature calls for common sense and awareness of its potential dangers as well as the great benefits it can offer. Adopting a more natural lifestyle does not mean that you can ignore the need for basic hygiene or fail to be alert to the particular vulnerabilities of your child. Neither the immune system nor the nerves and muscular coordination of the newborn baby are fully developed. All these continue to mature in the first few years of growth.

Even apparently healthy children can be suddenly overwhelmed by massive infections which may be beyond the resources of the self-healing mechanisms. This is where you may need the professional guidance of a registered naturopath or a doctor who can gauge the capabilities of the child so that he or she can prescribe accordingly.

The Principles

It was this common-sense approach to human ailments, based on observation and the use of natural resources available to them, which enabled the pioneers of naturopathic medicine to establish principles which have gained the seal of scientific credibility in modern times. Much of modern naturopathy was the mainstream of medical practice for ancient civilizations, such as those of the Romans and Greeks. The naturopathic physicians of the nineteenth and early twentieth centuries continued to make extensive use of water, sunlight, and dietary treatment to build vitality and encourage detoxification.

An important aspect of naturopathy is a recognition that poor health can arise from inadequate neutralization and elimination of the waste products from the body. As these accumulate they can inflict damage on the cells and irritate membranes, causing catarrh and inflammation, or skin rashes, among other problems. This toxic overload is now recognized as being due to the action of damaging compounds known as free radicals which are generated by the body from certain foods and also arise from chemicals in the environment and electromagnetic radiation.

Stimulating the functions of the eliminative organs, such as skin and bowels, is one way of reducing the effects of these compounds, but the stronger physical measures used for adults are not suitable for young children. Instead, simple diet changes may help the body's healing efforts and homoeopathic medicines can further act as a gentle catalyst to recovery.

Food Foundation

Healthy eating is one of the cornerstones of healthy rearing. Modern naturopaths have the advantage of the latest knowledge in nutritional biochemistry. Naturopathic advice may help you to determine the most suitable diets for your child's individual needs.

Educating Your Child's Palate

When it comes to eating, any child has her preferences and these can very quickly become for the least healthy foods. The formative years are an ideal opportunity to educate the child's palate. At this stage it is easier to introduce the preventive nutrition measures which naturopaths have advocated for generations and which are now becoming part of the health policy of authorities in many of the developing countries: increasing the amounts of fresh vegetables and fruit in the diet whilst reducing fats, salt and sugar. A diet of natural wholefoods not only provides essential nutrients for growth and repair but reduces the likelihood of cravings for sugary or salty foods.

> ### Juices
>
> *Juices are best prepared from fresh fruits or vegetables using a juicer/blender. Scrub or scrape the fruit or vegetable thoroughly and put through the juicer. You may use the juice alone or mixed with the pulp from the blender to prepare purées and soups.*
>
> *Juicing may be time-consuming and inconvenient, in which case you may use cartoned, canned, or bottled pure unsweetened juices such as pear, grape, apple, and pineapple (dilute by half with filtered water). Concentrated bottled juices may also be used and made up with filtered water.*

Encourage snacks, such as fresh fruits, vegetables, nuts, and seeds. Chewing a carrot or apple is also a valuable exercise in itself, encouraging the proper development of the facial bones and sinuses and stimulating the glands in the neck and throat.

Many canned and packaged foods, such as baked beans and breakfast cereals, contain added sugar, so try to obtain low-sugar or sugar-free versions.

Removing Anxiety

By working more closely with nature we have less to fear from the minor ailments we and our children all experience from time to time. The faster metabolism and greater vitality of children is reflected, not only in their activities and rumbustious behaviour, but also in their ailments. Most of the illnesses of childhood are acute and short-term.

Childhood fevers, rashes, catarrhal discharges, and diarrhoea are a manifestation of the body's defence at work. It is raising the level of activity as it fights off infection or deals with a toxic overload. In fact, all medical experts know that most minor ailments are self-limiting, that is, if left to take their course, they will usually get better. At most, a herbal or homoeopathic remedy may be all that is required to assist the healing process.

As you get to know your child's physiology, you will be able to judge when his or her system is able to carry the ailment through to recovery and when some assistance and control is necessary.

There may be times when you need to seek professional advice from a naturopath about your child's health. When might you do this, and what might you expect?

The Naturopathic Consultation

You might need to consult a registered naturopath if your baby has any persistent or recurrent health problems. Digestive troubles, skin rashes, respiratory disorders, and earaches are among the many children's ailments which are responsive to naturopathic treatment.

At the first consultation, the naturopath will ask you about your baby's symptoms and the sort of situations which aggravate or ameliorate them. The practitioner will also wish to know about the temperament of the child and the feeding and weaning pattern may also be relevant. Some children are more susceptible to catarrhal problems, such as glue ear, when weaned on to cow's-milk products.

Family history is also important. If you have a family history of asthma and eczema, for example, the naturopath may be able to give you effective guidance on ways of reducing your child's susceptibility to these often distressing disorders.

Once a case history is taken, a gentle examination is carried out and, when the practitioner has gained sufficient information about your baby's problems, he or she will discuss the measures you yourself may be able to take at home so that you can help mobilize the self-healing processes.

At Home: A Good Start in Life

The advantages of a more natural lifestyle from the very beginning are not just short-term ones – less infection, better nutrition, a more contented child – but probably longer-term as well. The naturally reared child has less likelihood of developing chronic disorders and allergies, and the probability of degenerative disorders such as arthritis and heart disease later in life is lessened.

Giving your child a good foundation in life is easier that you might imagine. It means applying some of the principles of naturopathy to your everyday life and surroundings. In and around your home you may not be able to make major and costly changes but it is worth thinking about some of the following and acting on them if you can.

Radiation

Electromagnetic radiation is a growing health concern as many modern appliances, including computers, TV sets, and microwave ovens, are a source of wavelengths which are not compatible with the human energy field. Most of us can cope perfectly well with the low levels of radiation they emit, but for a few vulnerable individuals, especially the very young whose cells are multiplying to form vital nervous and other tissues, they can be an added stress. Ensure that the backs of TV sets and microwave ovens are not pointing (even through a wall) towards an area where your children sleep or play. Check the microwave regularly for broken or damaged door seals. You can obtain special testing devices for this.

Ration the amount of time your young child spends watching TV. This is particularly important in the formative years when children need the stimulation of all their senses through play rather than the passive two-dimensional sound and vision offerings of TV.

Don't be in a hurry to introduce your child to computers; there are important skills to be learned from mental arithmetic, counting on the fingers and an abacus!

Ventilation

Keep all regularly used areas of the house well ventilated. Bedrooms, in particular, should always have a window open at night.

Light

Natural light is essential to good health because it has a full spectrum of waves which are compatible with our body's frequencies.

Artificial light, particularly from fluorescent tubes, does not have this. If you have fluorescent tubes in any part of your house, such as the kitchen or bathroom, consider changing them to the full-spectrum tubes which are closer to natural daylight. These cost a little more but give a better light and last much longer.

The traditional practice of putting babies to sleep in the open air, suitably protected from direct sunlight, is not without its value, and regular outdoor activities should be encouraged for every child.

Dealing With a Crisis

When your child has an acute ailment, whether it be a skin rash, diarrhoea, or catarrhal infection, adjustment of her diet may help the process of recovery. Resting the physiology by restricting food intake allows the body to direct more of its energies to detoxification and healing.

If the child is feverish she will instinctively stop eating, so recognize the wisdom of the body and give plenty of fluids, in the form of water or fruit juices. These will assist the detoxification mechanism without placing too much of a burden on the digestion. Generally, it is not advisable to allow very young children to fast for more than a day or two, but if any feverish disorder continues for more than twenty-four hours you should, in any case, seek professional help.

Dietary Treatment for Acute Ailments
While Breast-feeding

The regular feeds should still be given but the lactating mother should take care with her own diet. Exclude sugar, refined carbohydrate, meat, coffee, tea and cow's-milk products.

If you are weaning on to bottle feeds, change the milk feeds to fruit or vegetable juices for a few days.

With solids, avoid giving any milk, meat, or starch-based preparations for several days. Instead, use puréed vegetables and fruits. As symptoms improve, introduce cereals such as rice or millet.

After Weaning

Older infants may be given fresh raw fruit, raw vegetables, or steamed vegetables in a form which is acceptable to them. Mixed vegetables can be used in soups, which may be flavoured with a savoury spread or Miso. Maintain a non-dairy vegetarian diet for at least one week after recovery.

Biochemic Tissue Salts

The chemistry of life – or biochemistry – features a group of a dozen remedies known as tissue salts. Recommendations for biochemic tissue salts are made as part of the naturopathic treatment for a number of disorders, though you will not need them if you are using homoeopathic remedies. The biochemic remedies, however, are often more convenient for young children as their cellules dissolve very easily and the indications cover a broader spectrum of symptoms.

Hydrotherapy

Hydrotherapy is the use of water to promote the natural healing functions of the body. It may be used internally, as enemas. More usually, however, it is applied externally, as baths, sprays, or compresses.

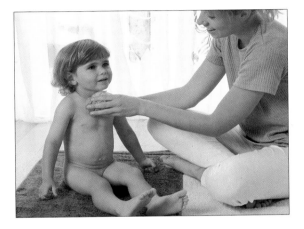

Sponging

Sponging with cool or tepid water helps to encourage skin function and regulate temperature, especially in feverish illnesses. For very young babies, avoid sharp temperature contrasts, and bathe the extremities only. The main objective is gently to increase skin function and balance circulation. At about one year you may apply water to the trunk, paying particular attention to the spinal areas at the back of the neck and between the shoulders in feverish cases.

Fomentations

Fomentations are short-term applications of cloths wrung out in hot or cold water. Apply two or three thicknesses to the affected area and use for children aged eighteen months or older. Avoid extremes of temperature.

Above. *Make the applications with a damp sponge or a soft flannel. Bathe for two or three minutes only and repeat as necessary at half to one hour intervals, or two or three times daily in less severe cases.*

Right. *Alternate warm cloths with cold, applying the warm for about two minutes and the cold for 30–45 seconds. Only hot fomentations may be used for asthma or abdominal discomfort. Repeat the application every five minutes.*

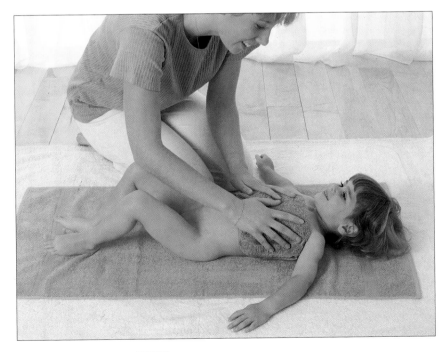

Compresses

At eighteen months to two years onwards, the amenable child may be willing to take a cold compress to the throat and round the waist. Ignore initial protests but be reassuring, and check that the compresses are starting to warm up after half an hour by slipping two fingers between the skin and the compress. If the compress remains cold or clammy after an hour, the cloth may be too damp or the child's vitality insufficient. Remove it and dry the skin, then wrap the child warmly.

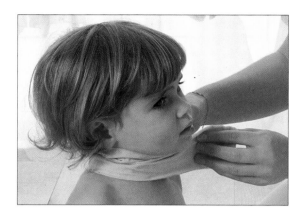

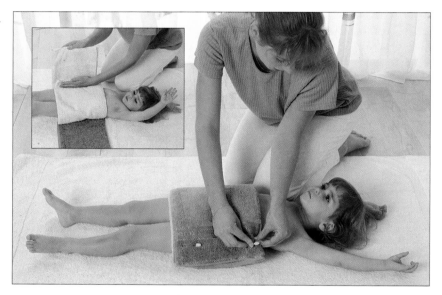

Above. *A handkerchief should be rinsed in cold tap water and well squeezed out. Fold lengthways and wrap around the child's throat. Cover the handkerchief with a small scarf.*

Left. *The waist compress, using a strip of sheet or thin hand towel, should be wrapped around the trunk from waist to groin. Cover with a thicker towel, folded double, and fasten with safety pins.*

Acupressure Points

Acupressure is an ancient oriental massage technique, with a system of pressure points that correspond to acupuncture points. It is thought to be a forerunner of acupuncture, using firm thumb or fingertip pressure rather than needles. Like acupuncture, it is used to balance the flow of *Ch'i*, or energy, through the body. It is largely a system of relieving symptoms, but is said to improve the body's own healing powers.

Right. *To maintain pressure, a small pebble can be held in place with a sticking plaster. The point shown here relates to vomiting, for example as caused by travel sickness. In the event of nausea, gently increase pressure.*

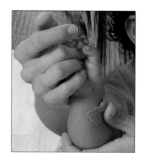

The Ragdoll Relaxation Routine

Good physical relaxation helps to reduce overexcitability and hyperactivity. Young children have not yet developed sufficient awareness of their bodies or control of their breathing to be able to respond to techniques which work for adults, but the following game may help to calm them a little. Try it after great excitement and before bedtime.

Find a comfortable space on the floor or a bed with a little support for the neck. The child should lie on her back with legs straight and hands just touching across her middle. Now she should breathe in deeply, and out with a sigh, trying all the while to be a rag doll. Breathe in and sigh out … and sag.

Right. *Say to the child, 'Think of your arms and let them flop'. Test her arms by lifting gently and dropping them on the bed.*

Below. *Say, 'Let's see if your legs are like a rag doll's'. She should breathe out as her legs go floppy.*

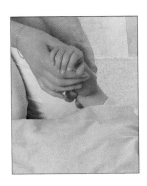

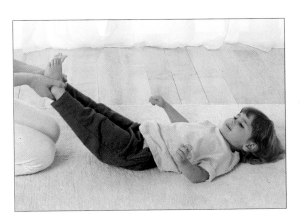

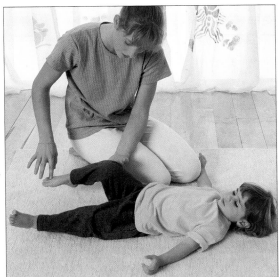

Above. *Gently test the legs to see if they swing from the hips.*

Right. *Let the head and body flop, while the child pretends they are a pat of butter melting in the sun. On the count of three she should breathe out and feel her whole body go floppy.*

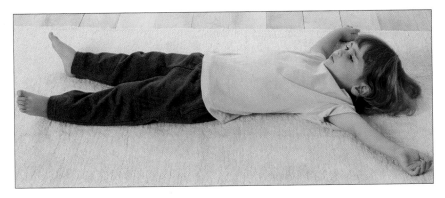

15

Massage

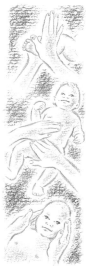

It has long been common practice to massage babies from birth in India, Africa, South America and Russia, to promote the development of strength and intelligence, coordination and balance, and to aid digestion and restful sleep. There are many positive effects attributed to massage, including improved circulation and breathing, decreased anxiety, heightened alertness, strengthening the immune system and stimulating digestion and elimination. Today in the Western world we are rediscovering the touch therapies and increasingly find scientific evidence and instinctive reasons for accepting them.

In the animal kingdom, many newborn are licked all over by the parent as soon as they are delivered. In many cases, this is a literal 'licking into shape' as the stimulus from the tongue encourages the functions necessary for survival, particularly the respiratory system, to start up independently.

The Principles

Massage is an ancient art of healing that has been practised for many centuries in different cultures around the world. Earliest medical records from ancient Egypt, India and China describe massage being recommended for restoring and maintaining good health. The Greeks and Romans used massage for recovery from injury and in preparation for feats of strength and often life-or-death competition in the arena.

It is very important, as various studies show, not to underestimate an infant's need for holding and touching. Scientists studying the skin and the importance of stimulation by touch have found this contact, even without nourishment, to be fundamental to human growth and development. Touch is the first of the human senses to develop and provides us with some of our most essential functions. It is through the skin, the largest organ of the body, that most of our external world is perceived, enabling us to learn about our environment and adjust to it.

In some South American cultures, the infant is transported in a sling across the mother's back as she sets about her routine at work or at home. The infant is in close contact with the parent at all times for the first six months. Studies now suggest that these practices provide strong motor and spatial stimulation as well as intense bonding with the parent.

Deprived of touch, an infant would become extremely apathetic and deeply miserable. There would be marked loss of appetite and listlessness in evidence. This condition could be observed among children in homes and hospitals in the United States, for example, as late as the 1940s.

It is now recognized that adults who have experienced abundant loving touch in infancy develop a strong sense of their identity and self-value, and are better able to handle emotional trauma as they are more psychologically confident and secure. It is in the earliest stages, the pre-verbal phase of development, that tactile stimulation through massage is of the most benefit, affecting all areas of our physical, mental and emotional health. As we age, our needs change though touch remains important in different ways.

Your Newborn Baby

The process of birth can be described as a series of shocks experienced by every newborn infant. It may also be considered your baby's first massage, as the passage through the birth canal, with the womb's strong contractions, begins to stimulate the infant's respiratory system. Birth is, without doubt, every bit as traumatic and exhausting for the infant as it is for the mother. Through the skin, virtually immediately after birth, with stroking, cuddling and suckling, the new mother can reassure and calm her baby and soon the shock of the birth will diminish. Without this assurance, without loving touch, the infant may fail to thrive and may go on to develop health problems.

Premature babies are often separated from the parents at birth and isolated in incubators. They receive less cuddling and touching than full-term infants and are more vulnerable. Dr Tiffany Field of the Mailman Center for Child Development at the University of Miami studied the effect of touch on these babies, comparing a group of premature infants who were regularly massaged with a group of isolated pre-term infants. The massaged group not only gained more weight but were more active and alert than the group not massaged. The study also revealed that, although the premature infants were tiny and appeared so fragile, the pressure of massage was very important. A firm touch proved more effective than a light stroking, the latter provoking a tickle response.

Clearly, loving touch is vital to a baby's growth. Breast-feeding provides the ideal opportunity to make loving contact. After birth, the suckling that takes place in the first few minutes is vital to the bonding between mother and child. The suckling reflex has functions important to the development of breathing and digestion as the breast replaces the placenta and umbilical cord as the baby's source of nourishment. The skin to skin contact of breast to baby's face acts to stimulate these reflexes and to contribute to the mother's milk production. For the new mother, this bonding intensifies the whole experience of motherhood and the pleasurable care of the infant as they become acquainted.

At Home

The attitude that you will spoil your baby if you pick him up no longer prevails, thankfully. Babies who are held cry less. Every time you pick up your baby you are communicating that you understand and care about your baby's needs. In the early days loving touch takes the form of cuddling, rocking and stroking the baby's head and back. Murmurings and lullabies, and talking to your baby in those special tones she already recognizes, all contribute to a deeper bonding. Simple stroking of your baby's body is enough in the early weeks.

As the baby grows and gains weight, the massage can be extended to a greater variety of strokes. You will soon come to know which

---

Contraindications for Massage Treatment

- *Do not massage when your baby has a raised temperature or fever.*
- *Do not massage unexplained lumps or bumps.*
- *Work around bruises.*
- *Do not massage when the child is likely to have any infectious illness.*

parts of the massage your baby likes best. When the massage is being enjoyed, there is plenty of eye contact between mother or father and child. It forms a communication that either parent can enjoy with their baby. In later months, the massage can include some simple exercises to strengthen the baby's muscles in preparation for the achievements of sitting, crawling and walking.

With the second or third child, it can be increasingly difficult to find time to spend alone with your new baby. The baby needs, of course, to fit in with the family's routine. Massaging the baby is an ideal way to make the most of your time alone with your baby and is relaxing and calming for you even when you may feel exhausted and not really in the mood. It will refresh and revitalize you as well as your baby.

The mother is not the only one who might want to massage the baby. Fathers have their own need to touch and bond with the new baby, as indeed does the baby wish to bond with father as well as mother. It is much more usual these days for the father to be closely involved with the pregnancy and birth of his child. The traditional male role has softened and 'new man' contributes more than ever before in care for the children. Fathers are much less embarrassed to be seen cuddling and kissing their children as the emotional barriers come down. Later on, that contact is shown in the form of rough-and-tumble play, particularly with boys and their fathers. Learning to massage the baby is, without doubt, a valuable way for fathers to spend that special time with the baby.

Older children, too, can see the baby being massaged and may want to help. This is an excellent way of easing sibling jealousies and may contribute to an easier acceptance and gentler handling of the new arrival if they are

---

Do's and Don'ts

A few vital points to remember when massaging your baby:

1 *The room must be very warm. Naked babies lose body heat very quickly.*
2 *Your fingernails should be short.*
3 *Until you are more practised and comfortable, make your first massages suit your mood. It is best to be as calm and relaxed as possible yourself. Later on, when into a more varied massage routine, you may find this makes you feel better, too.*
4 *The baby should not be too hungry, nor have just been fed. Allow at least half an hour to one hour before starting to massage.*
5 *Morning or evening, before or after the bath, when to massage depends entirely on you and your baby.*
6 *Use a light, natural oil (almond, coconut or an odourless vegetable oil). This should be warmed in your hands before applying to the baby.*
7 *Have a towel and nappy ready.*

---

able to participate. The father and the other children will all feel more confident and more involved with the new baby.

Essentially, there are no contraindications to baby massage other than those mentioned on page 17. Continuing studies show that massage helps alleviate many common childhood complaints. It can promote more restful sleep and a calmer awake time. It can also relieve digestive gas and constipation and may be of great benefit to colicky babies.

Above all, massaging your baby is fun. The pleasure and delight exhibited by mothers massaging their babies and the happy responses of the babies are a joy to behold. For a short while, nothing else exists and both participants are sharing love, trust and understanding through the power of touch.

Positions for Massage

While your baby is small it is possible to massage her on your lap. The best position of all is to make skin to skin contact with your baby's body on your bare legs. Alternatively, use a baby-changing console at a comfortable height. Lay a towel over the changing mat and massage the baby, ensuring that you are not stooped over her in any way that will cause you backache.

Effleurage is the stroke usually employed in baby massage for the very young. This is a gliding stroke using the fingers or the whole hand. Remember your touch needs to be quite firm to avoid tickling.

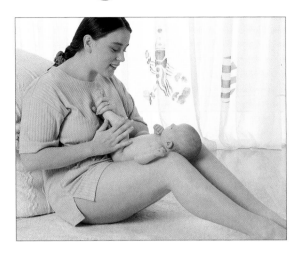

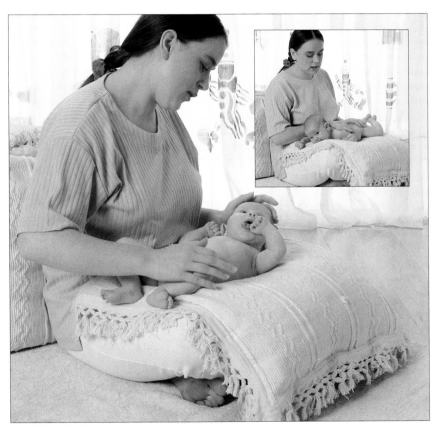

Above. *With very small babies, try sitting against the wall or a chair to support your back, with your knees raised in front of you. This allows you to maintain reassuring eye contact and observe the baby's reactions.*

Left. *You may prefer to sit cross-legged with a pillow or cushion over your knees to rest your baby on. It may be a good idea to place a towel over the pillow if you are using oil, to protect it from the inevitable 'accidents' since the baby will not be wearing any nappy. You can massage your baby's front first, then turn her over and massage her back (see inset).*

Aromatherapy

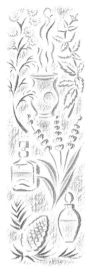

Aromatherapy is the modern-day practice of using deliciously fragrant oils extracted from aromatic plants for healing and general health purposes. Essential oils are taken from aromatic plants and trees whose healing and cosmetic properties have been known and used since ancient times.

Children can benefit from aromatherapy as much as adults. Babies and young children are very receptive to smell and will respond quickly to any treatment with essential oils. Aromatherapy combines wonderful scents with the power of touch and healing. The oils can safely soothe away aches and pains, saving the need for prescriptive medicines and helping the baby to sleep. When used in skin care they will help keep her skin sweet-smelling and free from the bacteria that cause nappy rash. They can boost her immune system and help her to grow strong, and should she be unwell, a few drops of a soothing oil vaporizing in her room will calm and comfort her, help keep her environment fresh-smelling and germ-free and restore her health.

The Principles

As well as their exquisite perfumes, essential oils are a mix of complex chemicals. Each oil has its own unique and individual set of therapeutic properties. When inhaled, or absorbed through the skin during massage, bathing, or in skin-care products, it is these properties that are readily accepted and used by the body to ease aches and discomforts, fight infection, soothe tension and maintain a healthy and supple skin.

Aromatic oils have been used for many thousands of years all over the world for medicinal purposes. Essential oils enter the body through the skin and by being inhaled. Our sense of smell has a powerful effect on us. Certain odours or scents produce an immediate psychological and physiological response. The nervous system of newborn babies is highly developed; their acute sense of smell can detect the odour of milk in their mother's breast and will stimulate their need for nourishment and survival. And, from a few weeks old, the baby will be able to recognize her mother's individual smell irrespective of whether she is breast-feeding or bottle-fed.

Essential oils are probably best known for their use in aromatherapy massage, but they also penetrate through the skin's surface when used in the bath, or in compresses and skin-care products. Their tiny molecular structure is able to pass through the hair follicles and diffuse into the bloodstream and cellular fluids. Depending on the amount of body fat, essential oils can take anything from 20 minutes to several hours to be absorbed. In a baby or small child they are absorbed very rapidly, usually within 15 minutes. The oils also act locally on the area they are being massaged into, so that a baby with colic or teething pains, for example, can be soothed quite quickly with a massage oil containing chamomile.

Following pregnancy, many women feel tired and experience minor health problems. Aromatic baths can relieve fatigue, aches and pains, and encourage restful sleep. Gentle massage using essential oils can aid relaxation, help the circulation and lower high blood pressure. Using essential oils during labour for pain relief will ensure that both mother and baby are alert after the birth and feeling well enough to get to know one another, instead of suffering the after effects of drugs.

The Consultation

If you are unsure about what oils to use for your child, or if she has epilepsy, eczema, very sensitive skin or any allergies, it is best to consult an aromatherapist before using any essential oils. Not all aromatherapists treat children or, indeed, adults with ailments. For any health-related problem, it is advisable to seek out an holistic aromatherapist. Aromatherapists who practise in beauty salons, department stores or health clubs are likely to be beauticians who have done a course in aromatherapy massage. This is not healing aromatherapy. They will not usually have the expertise or experience to deal with children's problems.

To find a good practitioner, contact a professional aromatherapy organization and ask for a list of qualified practitioners who have expertise in treating children (*see page 157 for addresses of organizations*). Your health visitor may be able to recommend an aromatherapist – good therapists are usually well known.

Fees vary considerably, depending on whom you consult. A child's consultation should be much less than the therapist's normal treatment fee.

During the consultation, you may be asked about the child's present condition (what has brought you to the therapist), the birth history and birth weight, the family history (any relevant illness that other family members suffer from), any family history of allergies, hay fever, or epilepsy (most important as some oils may not be suitable for use), any recurrent illness, and the child's eating and sleeping habits.

You will be advised on the management of your child's problem, and what oils to use at home. If she needs to be seen again, you will be given another appointment. You may be shown how to massage your baby to help with specific problems such as colic. Some aromatherapists make up essential oils, blends and skin creams in their treatment rooms. Others will write you out a treatment list of oils to purchase yourself.

Remember that aromatherapists are not doctors. If your child has a medical problem, see your doctor first for the correct diagnosis. Never discontinue any medicines that have been prescribed by your doctor for your baby.

Some essential oils are incompatible with homoeopathic medicines, so you will be advised not to use both of these therapies at the same time.

At Home

All essential oils are natural antiseptics, and some, for example lavender and tea tree, are also soothing and promote wound healing. It has been shown that a number of oils such as lemon, bergamot, eucalyptus and lavender can

---

Toxic Oils

These oils should never be used by anyone in aromatherapy as they have toxic properties:

armoise, arnica, baldo leaf, bitter almond, calamus, horseradish, jaborandi, leaf mustard, pennyroyal, rue, sassafras, savin, southernwood, tansy, thuja, wintergreen, wormwood.

kill airborne viruses, bacteria and fungi, and neutralize body odour. Some oils such as chamomile or sandalwood are analgesic or anti-inflammatory, their actions helping to relieve all types of discomfort.

Neroli and jasmine have anti-depressant properties and help to alleviate the tensions that lead to stress and mental fatigue. They have a generally calming and relaxing effect on the body. Other essential oils, for example rosemary and geranium, are refreshing, stimulating and invigorating, their actions being beneficial for some types of depression and during convalescence. They can also help to banish fatigue. Essential oils have other properties too: they are diuretic, decongestant and expectorant. In skin care, oils such as rose, lavender, mandarin and chamomile can help protect and maintain a healthy and supple skin. Roman chamomile is an oil you will turn to again and again. Known as the 'children's oil' because it is so mild, it has a wide variety of uses. Add 1–2 drops of chamomile to a warm bath to calm a fractious or overtired child. This will soothe teething pains, help heal nappy rash, ease the pain of colic, and enable your child to sleep.

How to Use the Oils
Aromatic Baths

Aromatic baths can be detoxifying and reviving when taken during the day, and calming, relaxing and soothing when taken in the evening. They can help relieve aches or other discomforts and encourage peaceful sleep.

Adults are advised not to bath or shower for a few hours after an aromatherapy massage to ensure that any oil on the skin is not washed off. Because oils are absorbed so quickly in children this does not apply to them.

Adults and Children Over Sixteen Years Add 3–8 drops of essential oil to a full warm bath. Mix the water around to disperse the drops. Relax and soak in the bath for 10–15 minutes.

Children Between Ten and Sixteen Years Dilute pure essential oils in 10–20ml of full fat milk (2–4 x 5ml spoonsful). Use goat's milk if the child is allergic to cow's milk. Count the drops into a bowl, add milk and stir; add to the bath.

Buying and Storing Essential Oils

• *Look for products that say 'Pure Essential Oil' and avoid those labelled 'aromatherapy oil'.*

• *Good-quality essential oils can be expensive, with their merits reflected in the cost.*

• *Don't buy oils that are all listed at the same price. Plants that have a high yield of essential oil, such as tea tree and lavender, are going to be much less expensive than the fragile flower oils like rose and jasmine. As a rough guide, 10ml of rose oil will cost twelve times as much as lavender oil. Some cheap essential oils may smell nice, but they will not have the same therapeutic effect desirable for aromatherapy, especially when treating children.*

• *Buy well-known makes from a reputable supplier, or preferably from an aromatherapist, who will be able to sell you very small quantities of the more expensive oils such as rose and jasmine.*

• *Buy oils in dark glass bottles, preferably with dropper inserts for easy measuring.*

• *Sunlight causes oil to deteriorate, so keep them in a cool, dark place.*

• *If making up massage oils at home use the blended oil within three months. Once added to carrier oils, essential oils last only three months. However, stored well out of the sun, a good-quality essential oil should last around two to three years. Some, such as sandalwood and myrrh, last even longer. Citrus oils however should be used within three months as they quickly go off.*

Children Aged Two to Five Years Add 1–2 drops of essential oil to milk. Don't dilute with carrier oils as it will make the bath slippery.

Babies Aged Three Months to Two Years Add 1 drop of essential oil to milk.

Babies Under Three Months Essential-oil baths are too strong for babies under three months.

Showers
Only suitable for adults, and children over ten.

Wash as normal. Then add 2–3 drops of essential oil to a wet sponge and rub over your body while you stand under the steamy warm water. Breathe in the aromatic vapours.

Foot Baths
For tired, aching feet, add 2–6 drops of essential oil to a bowl of water. Soak your feet for 10–20 minutes.

Compresses
A few drops of essential oil are added to either hot or cold water for a compress. This can be used with both adults and babies. Hot compresses treat muscular pains, teething, earache and period and labour pains; cold compresses are useful in the case of headache, sprains, swellings and minor wounds.

To 300ml of hot or cold water add 2–4 drops of essential oil. Lay a small cloth or towel on top of the water to pick up oils on the underside. Lay the cloth on the affected part. Cover with a dry towel and leave in place until the hot compress has cooled or the cold compress has warmed to body heat.

Essential Oils for Massage
For aromatherapy massage, essential oils are diluted in a carrier vegetable oil before being applied to the skin. The following carrier oils are the most suitable for use in pregnancy, post-natally and for babies: sweet almond oil, grapeseed oil, jojoba and calendula oil.

The aromatic massage relaxes muscles, improves circulation and skin tone, relieves pain, releases tension and hastens sleep. It can also help to lower blood pressure. Foot massage can re-energize the body and relieve tired aching legs.

Creating Your Own Atmosphere

Essential oils can be used to impart a relaxing or invigorating atmosphere, or to help dispel bacteria and remove unwanted smells.

A Bowl of Water	*To a bowl of warm water add 2–6 drops of essential oil. Leave to stand in the room to freshen the air.*
A Diffuser/ Vaporizer	*Follow the maker's instructions. The oil and water are added to a bowl, and the oil gently perfumes the air.*
Cotton Wool Balls	*Add 1–2 drops to each ball. Lodge behind a radiator or in your baby's room out of reach of older toddlers.*
A Plant Atomizer	*Fill an atomizer with 300ml of water and add 6–8 drops of essential oil. Shake well and spray around the room.*
A Burner	*Fill the top bowl of a burner with water and add 2–6 drops of essential oil. Burn the candle light for the desired time, then extinguish. Wash the bowl frequently to prevent a build-up of caramelized oils.*

Essential Oils for Babies Over Three Months

Essential oils suitable for babies' and children's baths and massage skin care:

neroli, rose, lavender, German chamomile (for rashes and sore skin), Roman chamomile, tangerine, mandarin and sandalwood.

Dilutions

For Adults Only (over sixteen years) Massage oils, using essential oils, are made up to a 2.5 per cent concentration (2.5 per cent of the total volume should be made up of essential oil).

Measure out the carrier oil in a container in millilitres, then add half the amount of drops as there are millilitres of carrier oil. For example, when using a 2.5 per cent concentration: to a 100ml carrier oil add 50 drops of essential oil; to a 50ml carrier oil add 25 drops of essential oil; to a 10ml carrier oil add 5 drops of essential oil.

Unless stated differently under a particular ailment in this book, use the following guide when making up oils for your baby.

Babies' and children's essential oils should be diluted to 0.5 per cent or less. Use a 5ml spoon as your guide:

For Babies over One Year use 0.5 per cent dilution – for example, add 1 drop of essential oil to 2 x 5ml spoonsful of carrier oil. For larger quantities, to 30ml of almond oil add 3 drops of essential oil.

For Babies under One Year use less – 1 drop of essential oil to 3 x 5ml spoonsful of carrier oil. For example, to 15ml of almond oil add 1 drop of essential oil; or to 30ml of almond oil add 2 drops of essential oil.

For an Everyday Massage Oil use just 2 drops of essential oil to 50ml carrier oil.

This amount of essential oil is quite sufficient for helping to keep the skin fresh and sweet smelling as well as helping to make your baby happy. It will just gently perfume the carrier oil. As with most herbal ingredients, more is not necessarily better.

During pregnancy and breast-feeding and if you have to make allowance for sensitive skin, use a 1 per cent dilution. The same applies to aromatherapy oils you may wish to use for older children, between ten and sixteen years of age. For example, if you are using a 1 per cent concentration: to 100ml carrier oil, add 25 drops of essential oil. To 50ml carrier oil you will need to add 12 drops of essential oil, and with 10ml carrier oil, 2 drops will be the maximum amount of any essential oil that you can add with safety.

Avoid These Oils When Pregnant

Some essential oils are too strong for the developing baby and others can stimulate menstruation. The following should not be used in early pregnancy; those shown in **bold** are best avoided altogether. Under any circumstances – even for non-pregnant women – they should only be used under guidance of a qualified aromatherapist, for treating specific ailments:

angelica, aniseed, *basil, camphor, cedarwood, cinnamon, clary sage, clove, fennel, hyssop, jasmine, juniper, lovage, marjoram, melissa, myrrh,* **oregano,** *parsley, peppermint, rosemary, sage, savory, Spanish and sweet marjoram, tarragon, thyme.*

Rosemary, sage, hyssop, and fennel should be avoided by anyone with epilepsy. Always consult an aromatherapist before using essential oils.

Aromatherapy Oils and Their Uses

Essential Oil	What It Does
Invigorating and Stimulating Essential Oils	
Cypress	Astringent, good for sluggish circulation
Eucalyptus	Helpful for respiratory problems and aching joints
Juniper	Stimulating to circulation; helpful to those tired and tense after work
Lemon	Astringent, toning and invigorating to circulation
Peppermint	Very strong. Good for aching limbs. Helpful for the fatigue that accompanies depression and baby blues
Rosemary	Invigorating. Excellent for fluid retention, cellulite, strains and sprains
Tea Tree	Stimulating and cleansing with anti-bacterial properties
Oils That Benefit the Emotions	
Geranium	Refreshing and uplifting. Good choice in an after-work reviving bath or shower for both parents
Mandarin	Calming, gentle and cheering. Relieves fatigue
Petitgrain	More refreshing than relaxing, but still shares some of neroli's soothing properties
Tangerine	Refreshing, uplifting and gentle. Suitable for children
Relaxing and Calming Essential Oils	
Bergamot	Good for those feeling depressed; smells good; liked by men
Chamomile	Very calming, a good choice for children
Clary Sage	Very relaxing. Excellent for tension, especially baby blues, but can be euphoric
Jasmine	Very relaxing and uplifting, again good for depression
Lavender	Relaxing and can help insomnia. Ideal for children
Neroli	Very relaxing and calming, especially for those suffering from stress and tension
Rose	Very feminine, relaxing and calming; a reassuring oil, good for babies and children
Sandalwood	Mentally relaxing. Sensuous qualities
Ylang Ylang	Relaxing and sensuous; especially good for nervous tension and anxiety

Herbalism

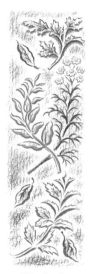

Medicinal plants are particularly well suited to baby and child care. They offer safe and gentle remedies and can be used both preventively and therapeutically for a wide range of common ailments from birth throughout infancy and childhood. Herbs are widely available for home use and can be employed by parents in a variety of ways which both enhance the health of their child and provide simple and effective treatment for childhood illnesses.

Herbal medicine is almost as old as human history – the earliest records are the Chinese treatises attributed to the Emperor around 2500 BC and known as the *Pen T'sqo*. The tradition of herbal use and the veneration of the medicinal value of plants are common to cultures all over the world. Herbal traditions have the benefit of modern research into the pharmacology and efficacy of herbs, which serves to prove that much of our ancestors' use of plant medicines was based on sound knowledge rather than magic and superstition. It is interesting that herbal medicine is still the main form of treatment among 85 per cent of the world's population.

The Principles

Herbal medicine has stood the test of time; centuries of use have proved not only its safety but also its efficacy. Because we have always used plants as foods and medicines, our bodies have adapted over thousands of years so that herbs are largely compatible with the chemistry of the human body.

Basic to herbal traditions of healing is the understanding that health is derived from a balance of natural forces in the body, and that illness occurs when this balance is disturbed. Another essential of herbalism is that the body has an inherent ability to regulate or heal itself, known as the 'vital force' (*Ch'i* or *Prana* in Chinese or Indian cultures), which herbal medicines have the ability to support and enhance.

Since the world of chemistry and science has focused its analytical eye on medicinal herbs, the pharmacological constituents of herbs have been widely assessed and their actions in the body analysed. We know that they contain ingredients such as volatile oils, alkaloids, saponins, glycosides and tannins, and that they can be diuretic, antispasmodic, anti-inflammatory, analgesic, immune enhancing, anti-microbial and so on. They operate in our bodies at a biochemical level, and yet their history and mythology have shown that they are capable of far more. While they provide us with valuable chemicals which support the functions of the body and its physical recovery, they also have healing powers that go beyond the physical to the realm of the 'vital force' – that invisible life energy that animates us on every level of existence, physical, emotional, mental and spiritual.

With the development of science and chemistry came the introduction into medicine of single active components which were isolated from plants to replace the use of whole plant medicines and then the manufacture of synthetic substances to mimic them. However, the modern herbalist still advocates the use of the whole plant as a gentler and safer form of treatment, as the active constituents on their own produce a more potent medicine bringing risks of side effects. In the whole herb, two main types of substance are found, both of which have an important part to play therapeutically. The active constituents are the primary healing agents, while the other, secondary, apparently less important agents play an essential role in determining how effective the primary agents will be, by rendering the body more or less receptive to their powers. Some of these 'synergistic' substances will make the active constituents more assimilable and readily available in the body, while others will buffer the action of more potent plant chemicals, thus preventing possible side effects. It is the natural combination of both types of plant substance that determines the healing power and safety of a herbal remedy.

The Consultation

Health depends on the harmony of body, mind, emotion and spirit and any imbalance or illness needs to be seen in relation to the child as a whole. In consultation, a medical herbalist will look at the presenting symptoms of the baby or child in relation to past illness or symptoms, their diet, environment and lifestyle – for example, whether she is or was breast-fed, relationships with parents and siblings, pollution in the home such as parents smoking, amounts of fresh air and exercise taken, and sleep patterns. The herbalist will also enquire about parents' and siblings' medical history, allergies in the family; any inoculation or drugs the child may have had, and the state of her general temperament and energy. Equipped with this information, the herbalist will proceed to advise on any necessary dietary and lifestyle changes and prescribe a mixture of herbs to address the underlying roots of illness and to help the body restore itself to health.

At Home With Your Baby

There are many ways in which we can use herbs in the home to benefit our children – as long as they interact with the body's chemistry in one way or another, they will exert their beneficial influence.

Taking Herbs Internally

We can eat herbs – breast-feeding mothers can add them to a whole variety of culinary delights, and their effect will be passed via the breast milk to the baby. Babies eating solids can be given foods prepared with them – parsley, oregano, rosemary and mint are familiar to all cooks – since such traditional culinary herbs contain a high proportion of volatile oils giving the benefit of anti-microbial and immune-enhancing effects.

We can also drink herbal teas. Breast-feeding mothers can take decoctions/infusions of required herbs, whose effect will likewise pass through to the baby. Babies can also drink dilute teas of most herbs – best given an ounce or so at a time before feeding.

Infusions These are made from the soft parts of herbs – flowers and leaves. For adults, use 25g (1oz) dried herb, or 50g (2oz) if fresh, to 1 part boiling water, or 1 teaspoon per cup. Cover and leave to infuse for 10–15 minutes. Strain. Drink immediately or store in an air-tight container for up to two days in the fridge. Use a quarter or half dosage for a baby or child, and give 3 times daily for chronic problems and 6 times for acute problems. An adult can drink a cupful at a time, and a baby or child can take anything up to this amount, depending on how much she will drink.

Decoctions The hard woody parts of plants (bark, seeds, nuts, roots and rhizomes) need greater heat to break down cell walls. So chop 25g (1oz) of the herb with a knife if fresh, or break it up into small pieces in a pestle and mortar if dried, and place in a stainless steel or enamel pot. Add just over 1 pint (570ml) of water; cover and simmer for 10–15 minutes. Strain and drink as infusions.

Syrups These are a very useful way to give medicines to babies and children because they taste more inviting. Mix 300g (12oz) of sugar into 1 pint of the required herbal infusion or decoction; heat until the sugar is dissolved; cool and bottle. Or weigh your infusion or decoction and add to it a quarter of its weight in honey. Heat slowly and stir till it begins to thicken. Strain off any scum; cool and bottle. Give half to 1 teaspoon for small babies and 1 dessertspoonful for children 3–6 times daily.

Tinctures These can be obtained from herbalists or herbal suppliers. They are concentrated alcoholic or glycerol extracts of herbs. Five to ten drops can be taken in water 3 times daily (or 6 times daily in acute problems) by children and 2–5 drops by babies.

Using Herbs Externally

The skin will absorb herbs – tiny capillaries lying under the surface will take their constituents into the bloodstream and then around the body. There are several ways you can use herbs in contact with the skin.

Herbal Baths An easy and pleasant way to take herbs is in the bath. You can hang a muslin bag of fresh or dried herbs over the hot tap, or add 1 pint of double (adult) strength infusion or decoction to the bath water. Alternatively, you can add dilute essential oils (1 drop per 5ml base oil) or herbal oils (*see below*) to the water. Soak for 10–15 minutes.

Hand and Foot Baths The hands and feet are sensitive areas and will easily absorb the herbs' constituents. Soak the child's feet in the herbal decoction/infusion for around 4 minutes, morning and evening.

Massage Dilute essential oils (1 drop per 5ml base oil) or herbal oils can be massaged into the feet, hands, back, and abdomen. This is a lovely relaxing way to have healing contact with your baby.

Herbal Oils Macerate finely chopped herbs, dried or fresh, in pure vegetable oil (almond, olive, walnut or avocado), on a sunny windowsill for two weeks. Stir daily. Press through a muslin bag and store the oil in a dark bottle away from direct sunlight.

Paste Dried herbs can be powdered in a pestle and mortar, and mixed with a little water into a paste. This can be applied to the umbilicus of a baby aged up to six months and stuck in place with two pieces of micropore. Leave for 2–4 hours and replace.

Creams and Ointment Tinctures, infusions, decoctions or dilute essential oils can be stirred into a base of aqueous cream and applied to the skin where required.

To make an ointment, macerate the required herb, as much as will go into three-quarters of a pint of olive oil. Add 50g (2oz) beeswax and melt together over a low heat in a bain-marie (double saucepan). Leave for two hours (or overnight). Press through a muslin bag, pour warm into clean jars. Leave to cool and use screw-top lids. Label.

Compresses Soak a clean cloth or flannel in a hot or cold infusion or decoction or a dilute tincture. Wring out and apply to the affected part – repeat several times for good effect.

Poultices Place the herb between two pieces of gauze and bind to the affected part with a cotton bandage. Use bruised fresh plants or powdered dried herbs mixed with a little water to make a paste.

Fresh Herbs Leaves or flowers or roots picked directly from the garden can be applied straight to the skin (after the leaves have been bruised or the root has been washed and cut open), for example a dock leaf to relieve nettle stings, lavender to relieve a minor burn, or plantain or marigold to staunch bleeding from a graze or cut.

Eye Baths The conjunctiva of the eye will absorb herbal extracts – use a decoction of chamomile and eyebright to bath inflamed eyes, or as a compress.

Inhalations The nose and the nerve endings lying in it provide another therapeutic pathway. Volatile oils initiate messages which are carried from the nasal receptors to the brain and at the same time they are breathed into the lungs where they are absorbed with oxygen into the bloodstream and thus circulated around the body. Aromatic herbal infusions or decoctions or a bowl of hot water with a few drops of essential oils can be used to steam a room. Alternatively oils can be dropped on to radiators, light bulbs (before the light is switched on) or pillows. Always make sure that the baby or child does not get them on her hands or in her eyes.

Useful Herbs

The following is a list of herbs which are useful for babies and children under three. You may want to keep a regular supply to hand.

Catnip, chamomile, cinnamon, cleavers, echinacea (cone flower), elder flower, garlic, ginger, ground ivy, lavender, lemon balm, lime flower, marigold, marshmallow, meadowsweet, mullein, nettles, plantain, thyme, yarrow.

Bach Flower Remedies

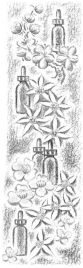

The Bach flower remedies are extremely simple and straightforward. They are ideal for home use in families as their application requires no lengthy training, simply an insight into the underlying causes of illness. Part of their beauty and simplicity is that you, as the parent, make your own diagnosis and treat accordingly with one or more remedies bought over the counter. The choice of flower remedy is decided on the basis of how you yourself perceive your child's need for treatment. This in turn depends on your understanding of her emotional state and mental attitude. The Bach flower remedies are concerned to cure not just the illness, but the whole patient.

The Principles

Dr Edward Bach (1886–1936), the founder of the Bach flower remedies, was a man of great compassion for all living things, particularly those in pain or distress. His desire to relieve suffering led him to train in medicine, at which he excelled, and in the first years of his practice he was a respected immunologist, pathologist and bacteriologist. However, he felt dissatisfied with medicine's palliative rather than curative effect on illness and was driven to continue his studies. His research as a bacteriologist led to his discovery of the relationship between the bacterial population of the gut and chronic illness, and the use of vaccines derived from

these bacteria. In 1919, working in the London Homoeopathic Hospital, he discovered the work and philosophy of Dr Samuel Hahnemann, the founder of homoeopathy, which echoed his own approach to medicine – the treatment of the person, not the disease. Dr Bach began to prepare his vaccines, now referred to as nosodes, homoeopathically and used them with great success. However, he still felt that he was working in the area of physical disease and not addressing the underlying causes. His understanding was that disease resulted from disharmony within, and negative thoughts and feelings, which were frequently manifested on a physical level. Stresses, such as fear, anxiety, panic, anger, intolerance and impatience, he saw put a strain on the individual, depleting general vitality along with resistance to disease.

Dr Bach had a great love of nature and intuitively understood that remedies for these unhappy thoughts and feelings were to be found among flowers, herbs and trees. So, at the height of his medical career, he left to spend the rest of his life travelling in Wales and southern England in search of such remedies to restore peace of mind and happiness, which he believed to be the essential nature of our being. During this time, he discovered thirty-eight plants which provided answers to much human suffering and which derived, with the exception of one, from the flowering part of these species.

Alone amidst nature, Dr Bach found that his intuition developed and his senses became more refined. His own intense experiences of physical and mental disharmony sometimes led him to find the right remedy in the fields or hills around him within a few days, for he could touch a flower with his hand or place it on his tongue and experience its healing effect on both mind and body. He also discovered that the early morning dew on plants exposed to sunlight had absorbed the properties of that plant, and far better than on those growing in the shade. So he devised a method of extracting the properties of the plants that anybody could employ and which would not damage the plant. The sun method involves floating the picked flower heads on spring water in a glass bowl. The bowl is placed on the ground near the parent plants and exposed to sunlight for a few hours, after which the flowers are removed carefully with a twig or leaf. The essence is then preserved by being poured into bottles half full of brandy. A boiling method involves placing the plant in an enamel pan of spring water and simmering it for half an hour. Once cool the essence is filtered and preserved in equal parts of brandy.

Since 1936, these flower remedies have been adopted with great success for a range of emotional and psychological problems. They are employed by many doctors and healthcare practitioners, but can also be obtained from most chemists and health food shops for application at home. Rescue Remedy, a combination of several flower remedies for use in emergencies, is also available.

The Consultation

As a parent using the Bach flower remedies you need, above all, an understanding of your child's state of mind. On this basis you can then make a diagnosis before simply buying the appropriate remedy over the counter. Generally, when a child is distressed emotionally or physically, you will be more aware of her negative aspects – and it might well be these that lead to the right choice of remedy. However, it is important also to bear in mind the positive aspects of your child's temperament and personality, albeit that they are more obvious when the child is well. It is often difficult balancing one's positive and negative sides; the remedies you choose should attempt to do this nonetheless.

At Home

From the literature that abounds on the Bach flower remedies, you will see that Dr Bach classified them as treating several different emotional or psychological states: fear, uncertainty, insufficient interest in present circumstances, loneliness, oversensitivity to outside influences and ideas, despondency or despair, and excessive care for the welfare of others.

When choosing your remedies you rarely need to give more than four together, once you have formed a clear picture of your child's problem; although, if necessary, you can use up to seven. The remedies you can buy over the counter are concentrated stock bottles of single remedies preserved in brandy and are supplied with instructions for use. You need to fill a 20–30ml (½–1fl oz) dropper bottle with spring water or boiled water and add 2–3 drops from the stock bottle of each remedy required. When giving the remedy to the child, place 2–4 drops of this directly under the tongue or add them to food or drink four times daily. The response will vary from one child to another. In acute states one would expect to see the child feel better soon, but with chronic problems the change will be more gradual.

All the Bach remedies are safe for babies and children, and there is no need for concern about overdosing. They can be taken with other medication and will not interfere with any different treatment.

Homoeopathy

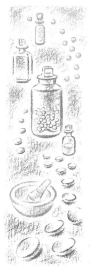

When you first meet your baby you will be struck by her softness and seeming vulnerability. You may feel that giving this perfect, finely tuned individual toxic chemicals is not the best solution for helping to achieve optimum health and longevity. Having a child can often be an emotionally turbulent time as well as being physically taxing. Homoeopathy is a gentle, holistic, natural form of medicine which can be used for a wide range of childhood ailments. It can be used safely and effectively both by the parents and the child and can help them achieve a happy and healthy symbiosis. Homoeopathy is well suited to this challenging time since it has the ability to treat both physical and emotional symptoms.

One of homoeopathy's great attractions is that it is easy to administer and can give quick relief. It is also free from side effects and is pleasant to take. In the case of one mother who developed mastitis with a fever, she found breast-feeding very painful and as a result her baby was hungry and fractious. She was convinced that she would have to give up breast-feeding. A few doses of the correct homoeopathic remedy, in her case Bryonia, eased her discomfort, cured the mastitis and meant that she could continue to breast-feed successfully. In another case a child was refusing to breast-feed because of thrush in her mouth. A few doses of borax cleared up the thrush and she began to feed again and thrive. Sometimes it is the parent who needs the treatment and sometimes it is the child. Whichever it is, neither of them will be harmed by it.

The Principles

Homoeopathy has been used for over two hundred years. It was formulated in 1796 by Samuel Hahnemann, a German doctor who had become disillusioned with the common practice of using toxic substances to heal people and who sought a gentler way of healing. He looked at conventional medicine and saw that it was based on the law of opposites. In other words, you use a medicine to make the body go into the opposite mode. For example, if you have a runny nose you would take a medicine to stop your nose from running. Conversely, in homoeopathy, if you choose a substance which in a healthy person would produce a runny nose, the person with a runny nose to whom it is administered would be cured. Hahnemann discovered that when this so-called 'similar' substance was used – similar in its ability to produce a symptom and therefore able to stimulate the body's own healing system into stopping the symptom – people healed gently, and permanently.

Homoeopathic remedies, the name given to the medicines used, are made from plants, minerals, animals and some diseased matter. These go through a process of dilution and shaking known as potentization, through which the substance's healing power is released and all harmful, toxic qualities are avoided. The remedy acts as a stimulant for the body to heal itself. All such remedies are easily available from homoeopaths, from homoeopathic pharmacies, and also from some large chemists.

As homoeopathy is an holistic form of healing there are no remedies for ailments, but rather for individuals who suffer particular symptoms in their own individual way. Their individuality is what leads the homoeopath to the correct remedy. Each remedy has its own characteristics, both emotional and physical, which have been discovered by testing them on healthy people until symptoms appear. It is from this body of knowledge that the homoeopath will draw, in his or her quest for each individual's appropriate remedy.

Using Homoeopathic Remedies

Remedies are generally sold in tablet form. The tablets are made from sugar of cow's milk, which is medicated with the remedy. Most over-the-counter remedies are hard tablets, which can be crushed between two sterilized spoons and given to a baby. Alternatively, you can buy the remedies as soft tablets from a homoeopathic pharmacy. These dissolve instantly on the tongue. Homoeopathic pharmacies also sell tiny poppy-seed granules, which are easy to give to babies.

Never touch with your fingers a remedy which you are giving to your child. Either put the remedy on her hand and let her give it to herself or crush it and feed it to her.

Always keep remedies in a cool, dark place and away from strong smells. In these conditions they will keep indefinitely.

Where possible, remedies should be given at least twenty minutes before or after food and drink. They should not be swallowed down but left to dissolve under the tongue. Certain substances are thought to antidote remedies so they should be avoided. These substances are: camphor, eucalyptus, menthol, coffee and peppermint. Mint in all its forms should be avoided, including toothpaste flavouring. Fennel toothpaste is a good alternative as are children's fruit toothpastes.

The strength or potency of a remedy is related to its dilution. The lower the dilution, the lower the potency number. Most commercially available remedies are sold in the 6 potency, which is fine for home prescribing. You can give up to six doses in six hours. Stop as soon as there is a change in the state of the illness or in the person. This is vital. If you go beyond a change you will over-stimulate the body and the person will get worse. This is unpleasant but not fatal and provided you stop the remedy at this point the body will rebalance itself and the person will improve again.

The Consultation

The first homoeopathic consultation for a child can take up to an hour. The homoeopath will take a detailed family history of illness in order to understand what inherited traits may be latent or manifest in the child. He or she will ask about the pregnancy and birth. Sometimes the baby will present a seemingly unaccountable state. The child may suddenly develop constipation and be very sleepy. On questioning the mother, the homoeopath may find she sustained a shock in pregnancy. This shock can transfer to the foetus and can manifest in the child later in life. On understanding the mother's pregnancy state and giving the appropriate remedy, in this case Opium, the homoeopath will resolve the baby's constipation and sleepiness. The homoeopath will also ask for details of the birth itself. Sometimes difficult births can lead to physical and emotional problems later on. If these are treated in childhood, they can be completely resolved.

With small babies case-taking is generally shorter and simpler than with toddlers. The homoeopath will rely partly on her or his own observations and partly on what the parents say. She or he will want to know a multitude of details about your baby. For example, whether she sweats and, if so, on which part of her body and when? Is she chilly or hot? What position does she sleep in? Is there any redness or any discharge? Does she smell in any way? Is there anything she is afraid of? Even very young babies will have their own individual fears and anxieties; some dislike being put down, others hate the dark, others prefer to be outdoors. All these factors will help the homoeopath make a prescription. Information about when an ailment started as well as the times of day or night when it is better or worse are all vital pieces of information.

The homoeopath will investigate all aspects of the child's being, from the food and drink she likes and dislikes to her sleeping patterns, dreams, bowel movements and moods.

In addition, the homoeopath will look at the complexity of the family in which the child is living, taking this into account when prescribing. Sibling jealousy, for example, is often seen in the consulting room and the appropriate remedy can help the child come to terms with this.

Using Homoeopathy with Your Baby

Homoeopathy can be used effectively and easily by you to treat everyday first-aid needs arising from injuries such as minor burns, bites, cuts and grazes, and less common events such as chickenpox. Follow the remedies given in Part Three (*see pages 135–56*).

If after six doses of your chosen remedy you can see no change – or sooner if recommended – you should lose no time in seeking advice from a qualified practitioner.

All these factors, when matched to the remedies discussed in the A–Z of conditions in Part Three, should help you in treating your child. Only give one remedy at a time for a particular problem.

Where there is no response from your treatment, it is important to get professional advice from a homoeopath without delay.

Observing Changes in Your Child

Always observe your child carefully, looking at what changes have taken place both emotionally and physically. Here is a checklist of things to look for:

Appetite	*Sudden cravings or dislikes for foods; increase or decrease in appetite*
Thirst	*Sudden cravings for hot or cold drinks; increase or decrease in thirst*

Skin	*Colour – pale, red, blue*
	Texture – dry, wet
	Sweat – present or absent;
	    smells or not;
	    profuse or scanty;
	    position of sweat, for example back of head, feet

Position	*Does a particular position relieve the complaint?*
Time of day	*When are the physical or mental symptoms better or worse?*
General	*What in general makes the child better or worse, for example being inside or outdoors, in a dark room, in a light room, in company or alone?*

Colour Therapy

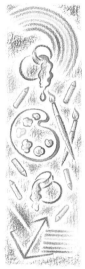

Colour therapy involves treating a baby, child or older person with colour rays in order to restore harmony to their body and mind. This can be done in several ways, described later in this section.

In order to produce a spectrum of colour, we need both the darkness and the light. This can be experienced during a storm when rays from the sun filter through dark clouds. The light rays are refracted by each tiny raindrop and produce, across the dark cloudy sky, a rainbow. Another way of experiencing this phenomenon is with a prism. If we place the edge of the prism against the bridge of our nose and look through it at the objects surrounding us, the prism will refract the light, causing a rainbow to appear around the edge of the objects.

All living things have their own rainbow surrounding and interpenetrating their form. This is true of stones, plants, animals and human beings. This wonderful symphony of constantly changing colour is known as the electromagnetic field or aura.

The Principles

The aura which surrounds a human is more evolved than that of animals and plants, and is ovoid in shape; the largest part being around the head, and the smallest part around and under the feet. The human aura is made up of seven layers, the first of these being the physical body. Each of these layers interpenetrates others and is filled with ever-changing colours. These changes depend on our state of health and our moods. How true are the expressions: 'red with anger' and 'green with envy'! When we become angry our aura turns a dark murky red, and when we are envious it turns a dark shade of green.

The colours in the aura also change with physical age. A newborn baby's aura contains very pale ethereal colours. As the baby develops, an abundance of red is seen to appear. At the other end of life, when a person has reached old age, there remains just a thin line of red in the aura, but a large amount of magenta is present around the body.

Disease manifests itself first in the aura and can be seen as a grey mass of accumulated energy. If this is not dealt with at this level, it will manifest as a symptom in the physical body. When treating a person with colour therapy, the aim is to disperse this accumulated mass of stagnant energy by re-introducing the correct colour frequency into their physical body and aura. With colour therapy, as with all complementary therapies, counselling must be given in order to find the cause of the problem. If it is a baby or young child that is being treated, then counselling will be directed at the parents. If the cause of the problem is not found, then the person will re-accumulate the energy as fast as the therapist tries to disperse it. An example could be of someone who continually hits their head against a wall. A therapist can apply colour to rid the bruising, but unless the person stops hitting their head on the wall, the bruising will not be healed. Another problem which can occur when only the symptom is dealt with is that the cause can manifest itself in another part of the body. A good example of this is eczema. Frequently this is treated with cortisone cream, which relieves the eczema, but the patient, many people believe, can then contract asthma.

Colour therapy is a very ancient form of healing which has been rediscovered. It involves administering the specified colour and complementary colour for the problem that the patient is presenting with. How often has it been said that when we are ill, we are 'off colour'. The ten colours most frequently used are: red, orange, gold, yellow, green, turquoise, blue, indigo, violet and magenta (*for these and their complementary colours, see below*).

Colour treatment can be administered either through a colour therapy instrument, which uses stained glass for filters, or through contact healing. Contact healing involves the therapist allowing her or his body to be the instrument through which colour is channelled to the patient. This method usually works better with young children and babies because it is much gentler, and the child also benefits from human contact.

The Consultation

When an infant is brought for treatment, the first question that is put to the parent is whether or not their doctor has been consulted. If not, then they will be advised to do so. Complementary practitioners, unless they are medically qualified, are not allowed to make a medical diagnosis. Details pertaining to the child will then be noted. These will include: name, address, date of birth, medical history, any drugs being administered and the baby's current state of health. When this has been completed, the therapist will discuss the baby with the parents prior to giving treatment.

The first part of the treatment involves making a colour-diagnostic spine chart. This will give the overall colour needed plus information on the general state of the infant. The

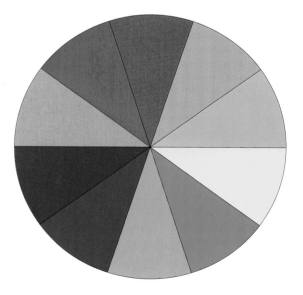

Left. *The ten colours used in colour therapy are demonstrated in this wheel. In treatment the complementary colour – directly opposite – is always used simultaneously.*

- Red – legs and feet
- Orange – abdomen
- Gold – solar plexus
- Yellow – nervous system
- Green – chest area
- Turquoise – chest and throat
- Blue – throat
- Indigo – eyes and ears
- Violet – head
- Magenta – higher consciousness

knowledge thus gained will be discussed with the parent and advice given on how the child can be helped at home in between treatments with the overall colour needed. This colour usually takes the form of clothing, to be worn by the baby herself, and also decor, which you can introduce into her bedroom.

The treatment involves, firstly, feeling and working with the aura to disperse any energy blockages that may be present, then laying one's hands over the infant's body to allow the appropriate colours to be channelled into it. If a very young baby is being treated, the therapist will usually hold the child on her or his lap. An older child would be asked to lie on a therapy couch. A parent is always encouraged to be with young children during treatment.

Treating infants with colour therapy also involves the parents. During a treatment session, information will be given on the colours most beneficial for the child and their use in both a preventive and holistic way. The exact number of treatments required cannot always be accurately assessed, depending largely on the disease and how long it has been present.

Partly because young children are not old enough to question its effectiveness, treating them with colour therapy can bring about wonderful results in a wide variety of conditions (*see below*).

At Home

For your infant to be treated with colour therapy, it is advisable, after a medical opinion has been sought, to get the help of a qualified therapist (*see Useful Addresses on page 157*).

Coloured Clothing

When treating at home, it is recommended that the colour be applied through clothes or by covering the infant with a piece of silk or cotton dyed with the appropriate colour. Natural fibres are used because synthetic material restricts the aura.

Solarized Cream

This is beneficial for skin complaints or localized infections. Place enough dermatological cream for one application into a small white container. Cover with a piece of yellow stained glass and leave in bright daylight for three hours before applying. Colours recommended for parental treatment of a baby are blue, yellow, turquoise, violet and pale pink. If clothing or material is used as a colour filter, the baby must wear white underneath or be naked.

Treating Common Conditions with Colour

Colour	Condition	How to Use
Blue	Temperature, fever, insomnia, asthma	Clothes or silk/cotton cover
Yellow	Skin complaints	Solarized cream
Turquoise	Weak immune system, colds, influenza Localized infection, cuts and grazes	Clothes or silk/cotton cover Solarized cream
Violet	Scalp complaints, bruising	Solarized cream
Rose pink	In need of comfort, love and contentment	Clothes or silk/cotton cover

Bates Eyesight Training

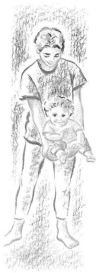

Sight is the principal means by which we are linked to the outside world. If the eyes are to fulfil this role in children they need to develop in a relaxed way, attuned to the rhythms of natural life. In our world, such a life has largely disappeared, replaced by reactive habits and adaptations to the pressures of daily affairs in a mechanized and technological society. Under these conditions, more help and support needs to be given to babies and children to permit relaxed, healthy development, which, for the eyes, can come through an understanding of the Bates method. The technique for this shows us how to be in particular harmony with our sight as well as with the other senses.

It is usually assumed by people who have vaguely heard of the Bates method that it largely consists of exercises to strengthen the eye muscles and is by implication disciplined and boring. This assumption is far from true: the Bates method is much broader, can be applied to most situations in life, and can be practised in many different ways.

It starts very simply, with becoming more aware of what we see and how we perceive the varied experiences of daily life. Exercises are used to focus the mind and reveal the interest in what is being seen right now. The more interesting sight can become, the more so the method's practice becomes; consequently the more possibilities there are for sight to improve by itself. Interest naturally resides in feeling, sensing and movement. With children this happens naturally through play. The parents' readiness to play with their child is crucial; it can be damaging if, for example, the mother is preoccupied, bored or irritable, and is unable to give her baby enough attention. It is important that parents work to maintain and improve their own visual perception.

Children soon become imprinted with the pattern of the world in which they are born and start to grow. If that world is stressed, so too will they tend to be. If, on the other hand, their surroundings are relaxed and interesting they should grow up likewise, with naturally good sight, focused and responsive. Sight, however, is more than sharp focus, important though this is. It is a mirror reflecting not only our surroundings but all that is inside us. For a parent to look into the eyes of a baby through glasses is like looking into a free world from the confines of a cage. The cage works well enough for daily routine, but can clamp shut on more vibrant impulses which should be encouraged since they are natural to life.

The Principles

The Bates method was developed at the turn of this century by Dr W. H. Bates, a distinguished American ophthalmologist. Its object was to improve sight and restore natural vision which had been lost through tension and resulting misuse of the eyes. Dr Bates first became aware that the sight can change for the better when he noticed that, among the great numbers of people he treated as an orthodox eye doctor, there were many cases in which the sight either recovered spontaneously or changed its form. Astonished by this apparent impossibility, he researched further, and found that poor sight can result from straining to see, and that this strain is primarily in the mind. It became clear that so long as the eye does not try to see, it responds normally. He realized that the remedy is not to avoid using the eyes, but to learn how to become free from strain. On the basis that anything which rests the mind will benefit the eyes, Bates evolved a way of re-learning to relax the mind and eyes, using a set of exercises developed for the purpose. In this way, the sight could be improved naturally and without effort, and adjusted according to its own rhythm.

The Consultation

The first consultation consists of gathering information, including evaluation of sight and perception, any medical diagnosis and treatment, the use of other complementary therapies, and information about daily life including work, interests, exercise, diet, sleep, and family and other relationships. The teacher should thus be able to help the client practise the Bates method to the best effect.

The initial consultation is modified for infants, since their sight cannot be tested directly. Instead, information is gathered from the parents, and the child's appearance and behaviour is observed.

The teacher will then show the first steps of the Bates system – to be memorized and practised by the parents at intervals during the day. These reveal, by explanation, demonstration and practice, how to let the eyes, the body and the mind relax, and how the eyes can remain relaxed while seeing. As tensions are released, so interest can encourage better sight. It is a

curious fact that often this cannot happen until the tensions that hinder it have themselves been identified.

The method is designed for adults and is adapted for children through an indirect approach. This includes play including ball games, stimulating interest, giving love and affection, listening without criticism, drawing and painting and generally drawing out confidence. With babies, the method will be greatly simplified and it may be more successful for the mother to aid the process by working on her own sight. It is certainly a good idea for her to learn relaxation, since her own tension and worry will hinder her baby's development.

The best way to find a competent teacher is to contact the Bates Association (*see Useful Addresses on page 157*). The Bates method can be incorporated into daily life by acquiring an interest in living sight, free from words and thoughts, through practising various exercises, a selection of which is given below.

At Home

For parents to provide the best support for their children's healthy development, they must encourage good sight. This should be as clear and relaxed as possible, without glasses, in order to give a natural pattern for the child to follow, and avoiding involuntary projection of parental stress.

The following simple programme can be adopted with benefit by parents, and taken up by children as part of their play:

Do your best to give yourself a clear period of time. Put a boundary around 15 to 30 minutes during which nobody may disturb you.

You can sit or recline in order to learn progressively how to relax. First, let the eyes be closed or palmed (*see Palming, page 41*). Then allow yourself to become aware of the other senses. Focus on sounds as you experience them, without naming or defining the source or type of sound. Listen, and after a short time re-focus on the sensations of contact by the skin with various textures; then successively on body warmth, body weight, the rise and fall of breathing, the sense of smell, muscular tensions, and body energies, completing with the visual awareness of darkness.

Now, as far as possible, allow all these senses to be present together. Feeling more relaxed, you can imagine that there is, inside, a quiet empty space into which light and colour can be welcomed effortlessly. Picture the colours that you like, and remember coloured things you have seen.

Leave your glasses off, or lenses out, as often as you can without straining, and always when practising to improve your sight.

Snapshots Continuing from relaxing with your eyes closed, prepare to open the eyes. Think of them as being like cameras. Open for one second, see the picture, and close for five seconds; see the picture develop and fade. Turn the head to take others, repeating many times.

Head Swing After a time, hold a finger in front of the nose and turn head and finger together, focusing on the fingernail. This will produce an awareness of movement. Then hold up the other hand. With fingers splayed, keep it still, while carrying on the previous movement and allowing your head to swing gently from left to right. This will help to integrate the two aspects of balanced sight: focus and awareness (*see below*).

Blinking Encourage your eyes to blink frequently and easily. This rests the eyes, cleans their surface, helps them shift their focus and stimulates their circulation.

Changing Focus To help focusing become more flexible, hold the forefinger of one hand in front of the nose, about nine inches away. Then look easily between your finger and a point in the distance for about thirty seconds. If your eyes are working together, when you look into the distance your finger should appear to be doubled.

Releasing Tension in Eye Movement Frequently, the eyes are stressed when making tracking movements – left and right and up and down – and the stress can be released by practising the kinesiology exercises 3 and 4 (*see pages 43–4*).

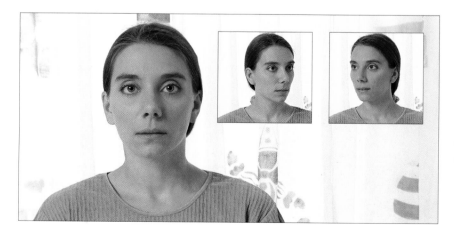

Left. *Head Swing. Sit upright in a chair and look straight ahead, keeping the eyes centred about your nose. Let the head swing softly from left to right, letting your focus move across the field of vision. This helps the sight to regain its natural movement and relaxes the eyes, face and neck.*

Harmonizing Left and Right The eyes work best as an integrated whole and this is assisted by harmonizing the left and right sides of the brain, and the right and left sides of the body. Do this by practising the cross crawl (*see kinesi-ology exercise 7, page 45*) and, in addition, by allowing the body to move to the left and right, the sight swinging across your field of vision.

Light and Sun Food for the eyes is light, which they need in order to remain healthy, and they can be fed whenever there is sunshine and a bright sky. Go outside and face the sun with closed eyes – never with them open. Turn the head first to the right and then to the left for up to a minute, after which the eyes need to palmed (*see below*).

Palming This is the basic way of resting and relaxing the eyes and the seeing mind. Sit with a straight back, resting the elbows on a cushion placed on a table. Cover, but do not touch, your closed eyes with the palms of the hands, with the fingers overlapping on the forehead. You

Below. *Palming. To relax your inner vision, first cushion your arms on a table so that – without touching them – your hands can cover your closed eyes.*

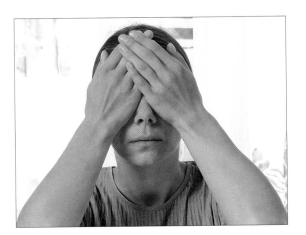

will feel warmth entering the eyes, and a restful darkness. Do not think about the eyes, but occupy your mind with something interesting. It is useful to awaken the memory: remember, visually, what you were doing an hour ago, or yesterday. It is also helpful to activate the imagination; try to foresee what you will be doing during the next hour, or tomorrow. Sight, memory and imagination are linked, and one will help the other.

Emotional Stress Release It is surprising to learn how much of what we see is stressful and upsetting. Such reactions can be relieved by using the ESR (*kinesiology exercise 2, see page 43*) while looking at what you don't like.

Having gone through the above sequence, you will find your eyes more at ease as you go about your daily affairs. To help this:
• Never strain to see – dodge whatever you find difficult.
• Don't stare – look for colours you like and things which interest you.
• Avoid day-dreaming – enjoy textures, and imagine you can touch whatever you see.
• Don't get bored – bring mobility to seeing by looking for or counting things, moving about and making comparisons.
• Never hurry – look at one thing at a time with full awareness.
• Try not to expect results – be aware of any movement in your field of vision at the same time as observing something in particular.

If you don't appear to be interested in seeing, palm and contemplate what it would be like to be without your sight. If that were so, what would you miss most? Picture your sight being restored, and marvel at the wonder of colour and light. Open your eyes and observe that you now experience relief and increased pleasure in seeing.

Kinesiology

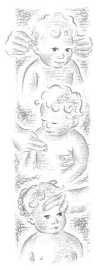

Kinesiology is ideal as a therapy for use with mothers and infants since it provides easy, safe and effective help in relieving distress and regaining balanced health. Prevention is better than cure, and kinesiology provides the means to practise this with benefit to mother, child and even the unborn baby. However, kinesiologists do not diagnose illness, or advise on medical conditions; instead they will recommend consultation with your family doctor where appropriate.

With the benefit of being simple, safe, and easy to understand, kinesiology is readily usable at home. It is important that mothers, both when pregnant and when nursing and bringing up their children, look after their own well-being. The baby, being totally dependent on the mother, will quickly be affected by changes in her state.

For the benefit of yourself and your family it may be a good idea to enrol in one of the available classes on the simple homecare practices that are a feature of kinesiology (*see Useful Addresses on page 157*).

The Principles

Kinesiology is the study of the movement of energy in the living body. It works through the unique instrument of muscle testing. This therapy was devised by Dr George Goodheart, an eminent American chiropractor, who in 1964 formulated the first applied kinesiology principles, starting with the observation that any muscle spasm is always linked to a weakness in its opponent muscle. This discovery opened the door to a new way of looking at the body and mind, and stimulated a flood of research which continues today and has resulted in the development of many branches of kinesiology, now spread through most parts of the world.

Following the first discoveries, it was found that all the muscles in the body are related to one or other internal organ and its associated acupuncture meridian. The performance and tone of muscles are influenced by the meridians and by various neurological switches: neuro-vasculars, neuro-lymphatics, spindle cells, and origin and insertion points, the stimulation of which will modify muscle response.

Kinesiology is based on the fact that the body never lies, and constantly expresses outside what is happening to it on the inside. Muscle testing is the means of learning how to read this universal body language and, in skilled hands, it becomes a uniquely flexible and accurate instrument, capable of distinguishing very subtle responses.

Various techniques are used to assess the body and mind according to a basic measure called the Triad of Health. There are two ways of testing. The first employs a series of specific muscle tests to assess body function energy. The second uses one reliably balanced muscle, called an indicator muscle, for determining the nature of a particular difficulty. The Triad of Health is formed by using the sides of an equilateral triangle to represent the three complementary aspects of structural factors, chemical factors and energy factors, which together form a balanced whole.

Once the assessment is complete, the usual way of balancing the body energy is achieved by gentle massage or touch of specific points, as revealed by testing. This may be strengthened by emotional stress release (see below) and nutritional advice, as well as specific exercises such as cross crawl (see page 45).

The Consultation

The best way to find a reliable and effective practitioner, apart from personal recommendation, is to contact one of the professional governing bodies listed at the end of the book.

The first consultation consists largely of taking the case history, including symptoms, illnesses, medical diagnoses and treatments, diet, digestion, activity, and emotions, and, with a baby or young child, details of the pregnancy, the birth and the first few months of life.

The kinesiologist will then make his assessment through muscle testing. With babies, infants and children, this will be done through a surrogate, since it cannot be carried out directly. It is energy that is being tested, via a conductor in the form of another human being; thus someone in a balanced state is tested while lightly touching the baby, in order to assess the infant's energy field. It is essential to include the baby's mother in any assessment as the baby will reflect any difficulties she may be suffering. The kinesiologist will then investigate the child's needs and how best to supply them, and will proceed with the balancing process. Finally, he or she will re-check any imbalances to confirm that they have been released. The kinesiologist may recommend simple forms of self-help for the mother to practise for her own and her child's benefit.

At Home

As the infant grows into a child, and her mental faculties develop, she can be helped through various problems with the aid of kinesiologies developed especially to overcome learning difficulties: Edu-Kinesthetics and One Brain, which contain many effective exercises such as Brain Gym, can be recommended. Touch for Health classes can also integrate the benefits of kinesiology into family life (see Useful Addresses on page 157).

Kinesiology offers many self-help methods to parents and children (see page 44 for techniques to use with children and page 47 for adult exercises). By spending a few minutes every day on the following simple exercises, the mother can help keep herself relaxed, energized, and in good health.

1 Water The body consists of 70 per cent water, and the proportion is higher still in the brain. Many mental and physiological processes depend on it, including the production of milk. It is essential, therefore, to drink plenty of water: 6–8 glasses of purified or spring water daily, and less for children according to size.

2 Emotional Stress Release Everybody feels emotional stress from time to time, and there will be plenty of it while bringing up children. It is not the emotion but the inability to digest it that is the problem, as if it became stuck in the stomach, and there fermented. Fortunately, there is an easy way to help release blocked emotions (see page 45). Frequently, the pain will subside, so that normal emotional 'digestion' can be resumed.

3 Polarity Switching All energy is polarized, not least in the body. It can frequently become confused or reversed, resulting in clumsiness, confusion or erratic thinking.

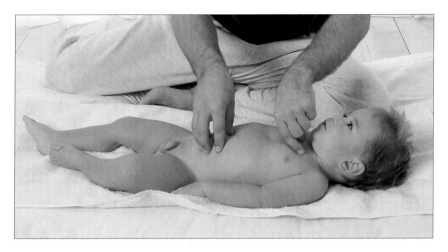

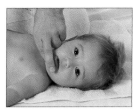

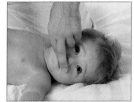

Right. *Emotional Stress Release. Use two fingers on each hand to touch lightly the bumpy parts of the child's forehead situated about one inch above the eyes; meanwhile re-experience the source of stress three times.*

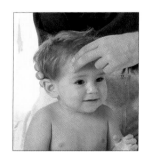

Above. *Polarity Switching. Energy can be rebalanced by placing all five fingertips of one hand around the navel (above left). With the thumb and two fingers of the other hand, rub two spots just under the collar bone and* on either side of the breast bone. Then, keeping all five fingertips in place around the navel, with two fingers rub just under the lower lip (top); and finally with two fingers rub just above the upper lip (above right).

4 Eye Strain The eyes, which need to work in unison while remaining relaxed and alert, are frequently subject to stress and easily become out of harmony and uncomfortable. They can be eased by adding the thought of a visual movement to the previous exercise, no. 3. With eyes closed, think of them swinging left and right (a); moving up and down (b); and stretching out and in (c).

5 Balanced Ears The ears resonate to sound and respond to balance, and are sensitive and easily disturbed. This exercise can improve hearing, balance and alertness. Children are more sensitive than adults, and this exercise, when performed on them, should be done with corresponding lightness.

Right. *The ears can be energized and restored to balance by gently but firmly uncurling and stretching outwards the outer fold of the ears. Do this three times, working down both ears at once from top to bottom.*

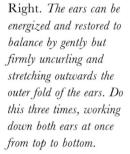

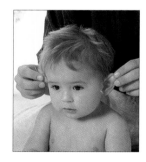

6 Yawning This is a natural reflex which draws energy to the brain, helps to ease cranial bones, and relaxes tension in the jaw muscles, while lubricating the eyes. Open the jaw wide and pretend to yawn, while massaging firmly any hard knotted muscles on and around the jaws. Repeat three times.

7 Cross Crawl The brain has two hemispheres which complement each other and control opposite sides of the body. A simple way to improve coordination in brain and body is to march vigorously on the spot, touching each knee in turn with the opposite hand. The effect is strengthened if meanwhile the eyes are slowly rotated one way and the other, several times.

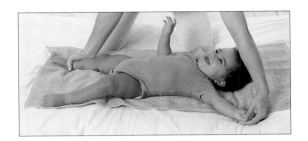

Above right and right. *Cross Crawl. By the crawling stage, integration of both brain hemispheres can be assisted by cross crawl. Your child will see this as great fun if it is treated as a game. The baby lies on her back, while her opposite limbs are moved towards each other, up to a dozen times. Repeat often, to help her with learning integrative movement.*

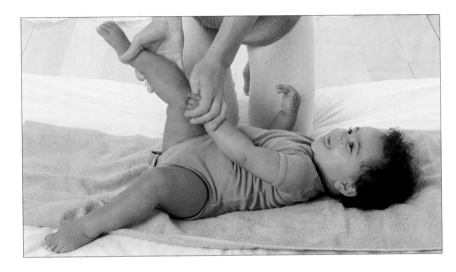

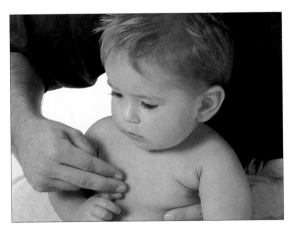

Above. *The thymus gland can be stimulated by tapping in a circle around the elevation in the middle of the upper part of the chest, in an anti-clockwise direction facing into the chest. Tap for about twenty seconds.*

8 Thymus Gland The thymus gland lies just beneath the upper part of the breastbone. It plays an important role in the immune system, especially in children. A healthy thymus is an essential sign of vitality.

9 Spiral Energy Energy emanates from our bodies, and flows through the body, crossing and recrossing the middle line in spiral patterns – or in figures of eight, according to how they are viewed. This flow passes all parts of the body, from biggest to smallest.

When put under stress, energy is easily disturbed, and can result in a disorientated sensation. It can be reharmonized by holding the palm of the left hand on the forehead and the palm of the right hand on the navel.

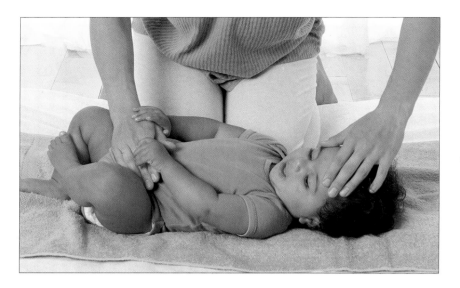

Left. *Spiral Energy. Lie the baby on her back, and place the thumb and two fingers of one hand (preferably your left) against the bumpy parts of her forehead. Touch the navel with two fingers of your other hand. Hold this position for half to one minute.*

10 Hyoid System The hyoid bone is located under the chin in the throat, and to it are attached ten different muscles, involved with chewing, speaking and movements of the tongue in general.

This area is deeply connected with speech, and with the stress arising from what we do and do not express. The resulting tension can be eased by gently tweaking the skin in a circle around the middle of the throat. Repeat this, once or twice.

Practising these exercises for a few minutes every day can bring great benefits to both parents and children. Nos. 2, 3, 5, 7, 8, 9 and 10 can be used on babies and infants provided a gentle touch is used.

Right. *Hyoid Gland. With the baby either lying down or sitting up against you, gently tweak the skin around her throat with a circular motion, at least two or three times.*

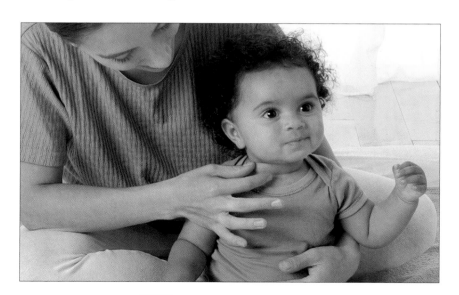

Self-help for Adults

A calm, relaxed parent is in every baby's interest. The feelings of fatigue and inadequacy that can follow childbirth will sometimes only surface months later. However, research has shown that regular exercise releases hormones which help greatly in reducing depression.

Right. *Cross Crawl. Stressed parents can relax by marching on the spot, ensuring that opposite arms and legs are raised together. The more vigorously this is done, the better energized you will feel. Try to vary the pattern, touching hands or elbows to knees, or hands to feet, as well as bending and straightening the limbs. While marching, rotate the eyes, clockwise then anticlockwise.*

Below. *Spiral Energy. This self-help exercise is designed to combat fatigue. It can be done standing up or lying down. Place one hand over your forehead with the thumb and two fingers resting on the frontal eminences. Lay the other hand on your abdomen, with two fingers resting on the navel. Maintain this position for one minute, and concentrate meanwhile on your breathing.*

Right. *To relieve tension, hold the emotional stress points while reviewing the problem. Lightly place two fingers of each hand against the forehead, one inch above the eyes.*

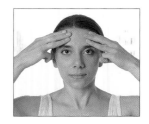

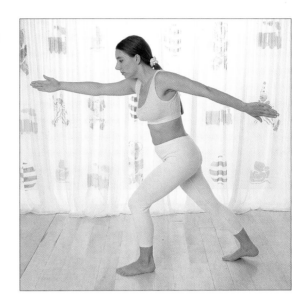

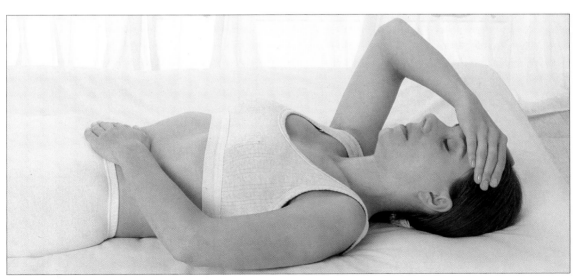

Sound Therapy

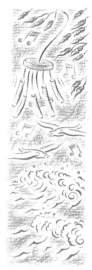

The whole of creation can be understood as a vast vibrational field, containing interactive patterns of unimaginable beauty and complexity. Such a vision moved many ancient philosophers to reflect on the 'music of the spheres', and inspired a longing to recover fragments of the grand design in composition and performance, not only through the art of music, but in architecture, design, dance and drama. An essential aspect of this understanding is that mankind, the measure of all things, is made in conformity to those same cosmic laws of harmony and proportion, laws which maintain the wellbeing of body, soul and spirit. It follows that disorders and diseases can be healed and prevented by music and by restoring emotional and physical harmony and integrity.

Modern scientific investigation seems to confirm the quintessence of this philosophy. All things can be perceived as vibrationary rates, as frequencies, as music.

The Principles

Hearing is the primary sense, being fully functional for many weeks before birth. Pre-birth auditory experience is important to our developing consciousness, and the unborn child responds in a very individualistic way to the sounds of the mother's body, especially her heartbeat. Undue stress or anxiety are thus conveyed from mother to baby. A completely stress-free life is an unrealistic notion however, and would deprive us of many vital stimuli; thus a balanced measure of stimulation and relaxation is the ideal for which to aim. During pregnancy, music can be a wonderful aid to relaxation and breathing exercises, and something to share with the listening unborn child. Do not however be tempted to turn up the music; no extra amplification is required, since the baby's hearing is extraordinarily acute and sensitive. Light, gentle sounds are the best way to stimulate reactions. There are many accounts of unborn children making their objections to certain composers, or certain styles of music, felt, with a timely kick. Brain scans have shown that of all the great composers' works, Mozart's music is the most effective at balancing the brain's two hemispheres.

Music can be a help in labour and many midwives encourage singing during contractions. Some mothers prefer to listen to tapes of music or natural sounds, such as birdsong or the sea. The use of tranquil and comforting music for the delivery itself is probably best, both for mother and baby. The choice of music is personal, of course, but it could well be based on the material which the baby seems to have enjoyed best while in the womb.

In the first year or eighteen months of life, there is much for your baby to learn, many skills of perception and recognition to acquire, and much of the unknown to be explored. The new arrival needs all the help, encouragement and support we can give. Every new sound the baby hears, causes rapid eye movement (REM) and stimulates the still-developing brain cells to make connections vital for the coordination of binocular vision, and the differentiation of information coming from the other senses. An environment of varied sounds, together with repetition from familiar voices speaking (or better still, singing) in recognized sound patterns, is a tremendous aid to the rapid development of awareness. It should be emphasized that it is a balance between the new and familiar that will provide the best auditory start in life. If all is new and strange, insecurity can, to some extent, close down the child's natural receptivity to sound; if all is repetition, then boredom and frustration will make the enormous task of learning seem even more difficult. As much as possible, the sounds should be introduced during physical contact between baby and adult as this develops trust and provides reassurance. So, for example, before you introduce the baby to a new piece of music, take her to you, perhaps at feeding time, so that you are physically close.

It follows that an environment in which a child is exposed to harsh, over-loud, frightening or aggressive sounds must be damaging. Trauma experienced at so critical a time of growth and development may set up life-long resistance to self-expression, and affect the ability to learn. Bear in mind that young children do not listen to words, as such; what is understood is the emotional content of a sound. They lack the ability, at first, to rationalize or process the fear, anger or disgust aroused by certain sounds, none of which can they avoid.

We do not live in a perfect world, and cannot always provide the ideal childhood or be model parents. But we can keep in mind the sensitivity of children, and take comfort from the fact that the voice cannot lie. Babies hear the truth of feeling behind our words, and the love we feel for them will nonetheless be heard and understood through our confusion, exhaustion and exasperation.

At Home

The singing of traditional nursery rhymes, and singing-games, are to be encouraged. Books of old favourites and modern songs are easily available from libraries and play-group leaders. Explore the possibilities afforded by any existing material, including tapes, videos, and 'singing' books, and don't be afraid to make up songs and sound games of your own; the words and music do not need to be polished works of art, nor must they be the same twice over. Improvise! Make songs for bath time, for nappy changes, favourite toys, meal times, the dog, the cat. Try to turn everyday activities, as well as special occasions, into musical fun. The act of singing brings the right and left hemispheres of the brain into balanced acitivity, making us more alive, and more happily vital. Songs are magic spells.

Draw your baby's attention to the sounds of the outside world – to the rain, the wind, the birds, animals, the sound of feet crunching on dry leaves, the voices of other children and grown-ups. Do not rely on radio and television to do this, for their sound frequencies are narrower and less vivid than the real thing.

Show your pleasure and award praise for recognition, and successful mimicry, for such play is essential to the development of speech and language. In order to acquire a language, a child must be able to recognize up to 300 pitch differences, quite apart from all the other elements of a 'mother tongue'.

Particularly useful instruments to buy are chime bars and glockenspiels, which come in various sizes and pitch-ranges. Begin by playing with a single sound, adding, one by one, the other notes to your repertoire, and making sure that each is special and regarded as a friend! Eventually all the sounds, and the spaces between them, will feel completely natural and can be reproduced spontaneously. Don't rush things. Allow the child to make musical discoveries in her own time, with your encouragement. Everything should be as much fun as possible. Significantly, we play musical instruments; we do not work them.

Participating in musical activities with other children is wonderfully liberating. If no suitable group can be found near home, you could consider starting one. Seek out and take advice from experienced music teachers by all means. But do not be afraid to take the initiative and lead by doing.

Simple 'one-two, one-two' rhythms are easiest for children in the first three years of life. Although listening to more involved rhythmic patterns will give pleasure, young children usually find difficulty in reproducing triple or compound times, at least until they reach their fifth year. Look for songs with 4/4, 2/8 and 2/4 time signatures. Melodies, too, should be

kept within the space of five notes for a beginning. Singing is a splendid breathing exercise in itself, and all songs should be combined, and memorized, with movements. In this way they become games, and these help to coordinate the eyes and ears with the arms and legs, balance, mind, emotions, body and memory.

Vary the mood; not all songs have to be jolly. Music has the mysterious power to take every mood and feeling and give it expression in a creative way. Make the most of it. Very young children can be taken into a more grown-up musical experience quite happily, if the musical content is neither frightening nor too loud. Children enjoy every kind of music, provided it doesn't go on for too long and it offers enough variety.

If you have musical instruments around, encourage supervised exploration and familiarity. Pianos and other keyboard instruments are fascinating to toddlers. Harmonicas, recorders, xylophones and tambourines are all easy and inexpensive instruments with which you and your baby can play.

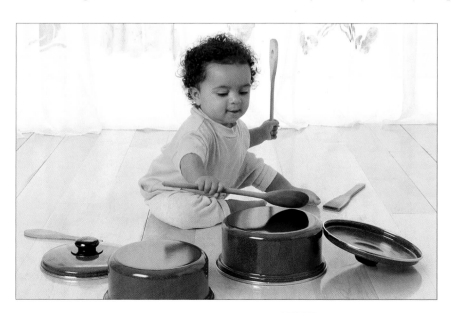

Left. *Play sound games with objects around the home; in particular the kitchen is likely to prove a treasure house of makeshift musical instruments. Spoons, for example, when tapped on china, glass, and metal, make intriguing musical sounds. If you vibrate a piece of taut string it will twang. Musical toys are readily available from the appropriate shops, but the home-made variety test ingenuity and are easier on the pocket.*

Alexander Technique

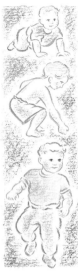

The Alexander technique can be invaluable to the parents of babies and small children, because it helps us understand how crucial it is to allow children to breathe, sit and stand, and grow as nature intended rather than forcing them into unnatural postures. It is important that you listen to your own instincts when making decisions on how to bring up your child, and the Alexander technique can help you develop the confidence to follow your own intuition rather than just the advice of others. It is a practical method which can help awareness of posture while breast-feeding, and can also show parents how to pick up and carry their baby with minimum back strain. It offers easier ways of pushing a pram, and with this knowledge you can also choose the best car seat or buggy so that your child maintains her good natural posture.

Using the Alexander technique helps you be more aware of balance, posture and coordination while performing all kinds of everyday actions. It brings into our conscious mind the tensions throughout our body that may previously have gone unnoticed. These tensions are often the root cause of many common ailments such as backache, headache, migraine, insomnia, arthritis, asthma and depression and, in babies and children, such conditions as asthma, colic, constipation, crying, hyperactivity, sleeplessness and tantrums. Posture is far more complex than just standing or sitting up straight. It can be described as the way in which we routinely support and balance our bodies against the pull of gravity. There are natural postural reflexes that organize this balance and coordination for us, provided we have the necessary degree of freedom and elasticity within our muscles in the first place.

The human body is an amazing anti-gravity mechanism, yet most of us unconsciously interfere with its natural workings, which is the main reason why millions of people suffer from back pain. Sometimes this is due to living in stressful conditions; at others it is the body's protest at having to cope with loads beyond its ability. Young mothers often develop bad backs and aching hips from carrying their baby. You can learn to avoid these problems through the Alexander technique. Your baby will benefit too, by imitating you rather than observing poor postural habits.

The Principles

The technique was developed at the turn of the last century by an Australian actor, Frederick Matthias Alexander, who kept losing his voice while reciting. He approached several doctors and voice trainers, but no one could help him solve his curious problem. Through years of experimentation in front of a mirror, Alexander eventually found that he was tensing his neck muscles unnecessarily, which directly affected his vocal cords. He was, in effect, stopping himself from speaking without realizing it. Even when Alexander found the answer to his problem it was not an easy task to eliminate the tension, because his way of reciting had become such an ingrained habit over the years. He eventually developed his technique to combat his own, and many other people's, tension problems. It consists of three main principles: sensory perception, inhibition and direction.

Faulty Sensory Perception

The first stumbling block that Alexander encountered was that his sense of feeling was unreliable; in other words, he was not in touch with his body. At no time before he observed himself in the mirror had he felt the tension in his neck, and even when he tried to release this tension he could see that he was tightening the muscles further. Alexander was surprised to see that he was not using his body as he had intended. At first he thought that this was his own personal idiosyncrasy; but when he started to teach other people his technique he soon discovered that they, too, were suffering from the same illusions. Many of us suffer with back pain; although we think we are standing up straight, we are in fact leaning slightly backwards or to one side, placing undue stress upon the lumbar spine.

Inhibition

To change our behaviour in any given situation, be it physical, psychological or emotional, we must first pause before reacting. Alexander called this inhibition. An example of this is when a cat stops before it pounces on its prey, in order to assess the situation – this procedure assures success nearly every time. Unlike cats, however, we tend to act and react without thinking about the consequences. Without this quality of 'inhibition', however, we cannot hope to change our postural habits, nor the way in which we live.

Direction

The third principle of the Alexander technique is the ability to direct attention to particular parts of the body, in order to become aware and to release tension. For example, if we have a shortened muscle which is affecting certain joints or interfering with our posture, we can direct our thoughts to that particular muscle and think of it lengthening. In doing so, we release any unwanted tension. Our thoughts can be shown to affect our posture, and we can use the mind to free our body as well as releasing past emotional traumas. The results are not only a more relaxed body but also an easier attitude to life. Many people feel happier and more contented after practising the Alexander technique. Their life often changes, from striving for the goals offered by the world, to one of fulfilment given by experiencing life in the present moment.

Learning the Technique

The Alexander technique is far-reaching in its effects, but it is at the same time simple and can be understood by anyone. The only requirements are patience and a willingness to learn about your own or your baby's body. By gradually becoming aware and letting go of tension, you will achieve a more relaxed muscular system. This will automatically relieve or prevent many aches and pains or common childhood problems.

During lessons, the teacher will help you to be aware of excessive tension in your muscles and to release it gently so that your body can work more efficiently as nature intended. This is done verbally or with the teacher's hands, which are used to lengthen the muscles. You will also be taught new ways of sitting, standing and moving that place less strain on your body, so that your attitude to life will often become more relaxed. Some people even describe the experience of a lesson as 'walking on air'! An Alexander session is usually carried out one-to-one, or on a mother-and-baby-to-teacher basis, and lasts approximately half an hour. You may need several lessons before you are ready to benefit from using the technique at home (*see Useful Addresses on page 157 for associations of qualified practitioners*).

At Home With Your Baby

Babies and young children roll and wiggle in an entirely flexible way; you rarely see small children with hunched shoulders or a back that is permanently out of alignment. If parents are prepared to contribute time and energy, the grace natural to young children can be maintained throughout their lives.

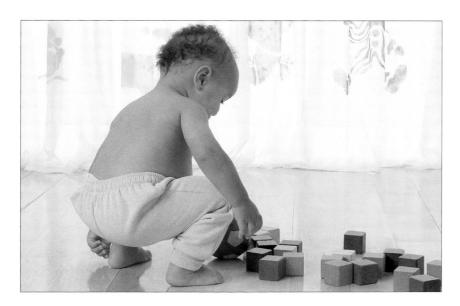

Left. *This child is using his body with a minimum of strain. Despite bending his ankle, hip and knee joints while squatting, he can maintain perfect balance indefinitely.*

Below. *The semi-supine position, when practised twenty minutes a day, can release muscular tension built up unnoticed during the arduous task of caring for babies and young children.*

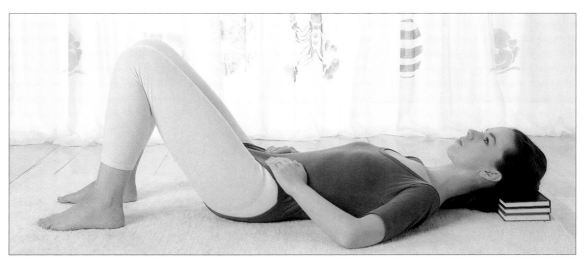

Osteopathy and Chiropractic

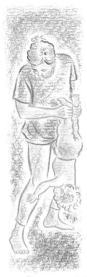

Osteopathy is generally perceived as a dramatic and forceful cracking of the bones of the spine – and as such may not be considered suitable for babies and young children. However, although these spinal manipulations are an important component, they are by no means the whole story. There are other essential aspects of osteopathy – softer and less dramatic – which are used as a matter of course in the day-to-day treatment of patients of all ages.

Osteopathic treatment is of particular value to babies because of the importance of a healthy balanced structural foundation on which your child's growth and development can be based – throughout infancy, childhood, and adulthood. Structural aberrations may be present from birth, from various different causes, and if treated early are more likely to respond rapidly and be resolved completely. Any imbalances and asymmetries may otherwise become part of the growth pattern, solidifying into the body's structure – and consequently impeding the function of the blood vessels and nerves which regulate our bodily workings.

Osteopathy was developed by Andrew Taylor Still, an American doctor, in the mid-nineteenth century. He, in fact, devised its principles primarily for the treatment of infectious diseases. Dr Still expanded his ideas to create a comprehensive system of manual medicine, aimed at treating a wide range of conditions and maintaining good health generally, on the basis that the integrity of the structure of the body is vital to its function.

Around the beginning of this century, in the United States, chiropractic was formed as an offshoot of osteopathy; and these days, while osteopathy may be widely practised elsewhere, in the United States a chiropractor is much easier to find than an osteopath.

The Principles

The essential principle that Still established was that structure and function are interrelated. In other words, if the structure is aberrant in any way, the body will not function effectively. If there is malfunction of any kind, equally it will affect the body's structure. Consequently there will always be a structural component through which that dysfunction can be identified, located and treated.

It is important to recognize that structure does not mean only the more solid parts of the bones and muscles, but also the softer components making up the body systems, including blood vessels, nerves, and all the tissues which in turn influence fluid flow and nerve supply.

The fundamental principles of osteopathy which follow from this are:
• that proper blood flow to each and every part of the body is needed for healthy function
• that proper nerve supply to every part of the body is likewise essential.

Ensuring the free flow of arterial supply, venous and lymphatic drainage and nerve supply, not only provides each part of the body with the nutrients, oxygen and drainage that it requires. It also ensures transport of the body's healing mechanisms, to enable it to deal with infections and other disorders and to allow proper repair following injury or illness.

In osteopathy therefore, the central aim is to establish a balanced, symmetrical and freely mobile structure within which the body's systems can function effectively.

This structural balance is achieved through the articulations and soft-tissue techniques of osteopathy. These ease restrictions – releasing tensions in the muscles, tendons, ligaments and other soft tissues of the body, and freeing the joints in the spine, hips, shoulders and elsewhere. In babies this is of course carried out very gently – massaging the muscles and soft tissues in a way that is comforting for the baby.

On a very gentle level there is also a branch of osteopathy known as cranial osteopathy. This is particularly suitable for babies, but is practised only by a small minority of osteopaths. It is essentially the same as craniosacral therapy and is dealt with under that heading in this book (*see pages 56–8*).

Chiropractic, started as an offshoot of osteopathy, developed at the beginning of this century with the intention of maintaining a treatment system with a more mechanical framework. It remains, for the most part, a more mechanically orientated approach, concentrating more on the treatment of the spine than the body as a whole. It also places greater emphasis on the more forceful manipulations of the spine and is therefore less suitable for babies and children.

The Consultation

An osteopath generally starts by taking a detailed case history. He or she will observe your baby's overall symmetry, both in structure and movement. You will probably be asked to undress your baby at least down to the nappy to enable a thorough examination. This should cover the whole body, with specific attention to any areas that are causing concern. The osteopath will explore each part of the body, testing mobility, feeling for tension or restriction. She or he then encourages the release of any tensions, through gentle massaging of the soft tissues of the joints.

Finding a Therapist

Although the principles of osteopathy can be applied readily to babies and young children, not many osteopaths use these more structural forms in treating them. Those who do treat babies tend to develop other approaches, particularly cranial osteopathy.

Your national organization will help you find a qualified osteopath who specifically treats babies (*see Useful Addresses on page 157*). Alternatively, you can seek a recommendation by word of mouth.

At Home

By following professional treatment you should be able to assist your baby's development. Ways in which this can be done include:
• encouraging mobility in restricted areas through gentle movements of limbs or body
• encouraging symmetrical limb movements
• favouring certain lying or sitting positions
• encouraging movement in parts of the body which are perhaps not fully used.

Every chance to massage your baby – in the bath, on the bed, while playing – is valuable (*see pages 16–19*). Encouraging a general flexibility and relaxation is always beneficial. Parents will soon learn to identify areas of tightness and can work on these to help them dissipate. Feedback from the parents to the osteopath can also be valuable.

Cranio-sacral Therapy

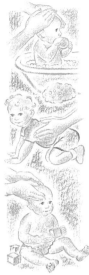

Cranio-sacral therapy is of relevance to babies for four principal reasons. Firstly, it is exceptionally gentle and non-invasive. Babies can be treated while asleep, or contentedly feeding. If they are awake, they generally appreciate this gentle soothing treatment, and tend to smile, gurgle, and settle down in response.

Secondly, the therapy is effective in treating many conditions which commonly affect babies, including some not readily treated by other means. These include colic and colic-like symptoms, poor sleep, persistent crying, feeding difficulties, restlessness, and hyperactivity. Craniosacral therapy is also effective in treating common ear infections, glue ear, and ENT problems, thereby removing the need for antibiotics and subsequent invasive treatment such as the insertion of grommets. It can also be helpful in minimizing the after effects of more serious infections such as meningitis.

Thirdly, through cranio-sacral therapy it is possible to identify at a very early age – and prevent the development of – conditions which otherwise might not manifest until years later. These include dyslexia, learning difficulties, autism, epilepsy, squint, poor coordination, and hyperactivity.

Ultimately, however, the most important aspect of cranio-sacral treatment for babies is providing a good start in life, by ironing out any restrictions, asymmetries or health problems at the earliest opportunity. These may have arisen from compression of the cranium, or other stresses due to a traumatic or difficult birth, from intra-uterine problems or through injuries or illnesses in early neonate life.

Ensuring a balanced healthy state through cranio-sacral therapy, sets up a positive basis on which the child can grow and develop. Specific restrictions and apparently minor abnormalities – generally not diagnosed or given importance – can be identified while still recent and amenable to treatment, and before they become fixed into the growth patterns. The soft malleable cranium and the rest of the body's structure rapidly harden and become set into their patterns (or asymmetries) during the first year or two of life. Minor asymmetries and restrictions can lead to debilitating conditions later on in the child's development. For example, colic symptoms often disappear at around three months old, but if the condition is left untreated it may predispose to duodenal ulcers, hiatus hernia or other disorders affecting the digestive system.

What is also important is that a baby who is happy, smiling, comfortable and well, gains a positive response from everyone she meets and a consequent positive outlook on life. A baby who is uncomfortable, crying, screaming and keeping her parents awake half the night gets a less encouraging response, even from her devoted but exhausted parents, and thus has a very different, less happy outlook and experience of the world. This again sets patterns for the future.

The principles underlying cranio-sacral therapy were first developed under the name of cranial osteopathy by an American osteopath, Dr William Sutherland, in the 1930s. Dr Sutherland started to teach his ideas on the cranio-sacral system to a small group of fellow osteopaths in the 1950s in the United States. Since then its effectiveness, particularly in areas not previously treated by other means, has lead to its rapid spread. Various others have expanded the principles outlined by Sutherland and the therapy continues to develop and progress.

The Principles

The cranio-sacral system consists of the membranes which surround the central nervous system (the brain and spinal cord), the bones of the cranium and sacrum which attach to these membranes, the fascia which radiates out from the membrane to all parts of the body, enveloping every nerve and nerve pathway, and the cerebro-spinal fluid – a vital substance transmitted from its reservoir within and around the central nervous system along neurological pathways to every structure throughout the body, carrying a potent healing energy.

All these structures pulsate in a symmetrical balanced motion, the cranial rhythm, reflected out to all parts of the body.

The free flow of fluid to every tissue in the body is essential. Blockage of fluid pathways will result in dysfunction and disease; release of restrictions will restore healthy function. Such blockage may result from injury, infection, inflammation, structural imbalance, muscular strain, emotional tension, or any disease.

Every injury, illness, stress or health problem leaves its mark on the body. The effects are reflected as disturbances of rhythm and symmetry in the cranio-sacral system, or as abnormal pulls and tensions within the body tissues. These can be identified, traced to their source and diagnosed by the cranio-sacral therapist. Similarly, balance and symmetry within the cranio-sacral system are reflected out to create balance and free unrestricted function to the rest of the body. The cranio-sacral therapist can restore balance, free mobility, free fluid flow and free energy flow and consequent healthy function not only to the affected area, but ultimately to the whole body.

The aims of cranio-sacral therapy can therefore be summarized as:
• release of any blockages impeding normal healthy function
• unravelling and disentangling tensions, compressions, adhesions and constrictions, which accumulate in the body as a result of injury, illness or stress
• ensuring the free flow of healing energy and body fluids (cerebro-spinal fluid, arterial blood, venous drainage, lymphatic drainage, *Ch'i*, *Prana*, and healing energy) to all parts of the body in order to bring the whole person into a state of balance and well-being in which all the body's systems (the nervous, immune, digestive, respiratory, cardio-vascular, hormonal, and musculo-skeletal systems) can operate at their optimum level.

Treatment consists of the practitioner placing his or her hands very gently on the body, identifying the areas of restriction or tension, and following the subtle internal pulls and twists manifested by the cranio-sacral system until points of resistance are encountered and released. The experience is generally comforting, creating a sense of well-being.

The Consultation

When a baby is brought for treatment, one priority is for the cranio-sacral therapist to create an harmonious relationship with her, since a contented child responds more positively to any form of treatment, and a relaxed cranio-sacral system will also be likely to cooperate more readily.

The therapist will generally take a detailed case history from the baby's parents, though much of the relevant information will emerge as treatment progresses, and the most significant information will be gained by what the therapist can feel in the baby's cranio-sacral system and body. There is no need to undress the baby (which is always appreciated by both baby and parent) since the patterns exhibited by the cranio-sacral system are easily felt through clothes, even several layers of nappy and babygrow.

Your baby can be treated in her mother's or father's arms, while asleep or feeding, or lying comfortably on a soft pillow.

There are also cranial osteopaths who practise in a similar way, but only around 10 per cent of osteopaths work on the cranium, and there is at present no qualification by which one can distinguish them (*for cranio-sacral therapists, see Useful Addresses on page 157*).

At Home

It is important for parents to be aware of the conditions which can be helped by cranio-sacral therapy, and in what circumstances. So many parents endure months, even years, of sleepless nights with crying, screaming, colicky babies, or are told to give countless courses of antibiotics which could be avoided.

Because cranio-sacral therapy requires such a subtle sensitivity, it cannot be readily applied by untrained parents. Given how delicate babies can be, it is best for treatment to be carried out by a skilled cranio-sacral therapist. Ideally, every baby would benefit from a comprehensive check by an experienced therapist at the earliest opportunity to identify any restrictions. Subsequent regular check-ups can be made throughout childhood to deal with ill-nesses and injuries as they occur. Most conditions can be quickly cured if they are treated early enough.

However, while actual treatment requires the highly developed sensitivity and skills of a cranio-sacral therapist, there are ways in which parents may be able to assist.

One of these is by getting your baby accustomed to being touched and stroked in the way that cranio-sacral therapists make contact. Stroke your baby very gently, using a butterfly touch and resting your hands lightly on her. This is particularly important on the head. Many babies will resent any contact on their head during treatment and may try to wriggle out of reach or push the practitioner's hands away. If they become used to this procedure at home with their parents, they will accept it more readily. It must be emphasized that the contact is extremely light and in no way is pressure exerted on your baby's head.

Once areas of tension and restriction have been identified, parents may be able to assist release by gently stroking and massaging each area. This is something that can be done on a day-to-day basis, in the bath, while changing, and during play.

Another way in which parents can help is by favouring certain positions for lying or sitting the baby. If patterns of asymmetry have been identified by a therapist, it may be helpful to lie your baby in certain ways in order to open up areas of tightness and restriction. This can be particularly relevant when the baby's neck has a tendency to turn one way or another. The parents can, again very gently, encourage gentle rotation of the neck in the opposite direction. No force should ever be applied, just a repeated persuasion of the body to a more balanced symmetrical state. Parents can also encourage more exercise of parts of the body which are not being fully used.

Movement and Dance

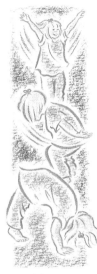

Creative play and movement games for fun and fitness are an essential part of your life with your new baby. They are needed to maintain the natural harmony of body and mind and to ward off complaints and disorders caused by anxiety, lack of exercise, confinement and boredom. The 'normal' baby has a tremendous need to move and wriggle about during her waking hours. A well baby, likewise, has enormous natural energy. As she grows, every waking moment is filled with increasingly intense and focused movement. Babies move intuitively and constantly, because every system of the body needs motion to function:

• Muscles need to be stretched and toned.

• Bones need to be strengthened.

• Breathing and circulation both have to be properly stimulated.

• Digestion, the nervous system and the lymphatic system all require movement in order to function efficiently.

For the growing, developing baby, after food, shelter and someone to love, nothing is more important than the time and space in which to move. The spontaneous movement of very young babies quickly becomes what we call 'movement play'. Their natural curiosity about themselves and everything around them is expressed in movement. It could be described as their one obsession. It is their means to understanding themselves and their rapidly changing, developing body and personality. It is the way in which they find out about the world around them. They learn to judge space, weight and distance, practising skills that will make them stronger, safer and more confident.

Babies and young children make physical contact as an important part of relating to others. They become 'social' beings, matching movement with emotion – 'hug you', 'go away' – and with other meaning.

Even very young children learn to choose, make decisions and organize themselves, and set their own pace and be in control of their own space as far as they are able. In our over-organized society and modern, fast way of life, it is sometimes too easy to overlook this vital need for creative movement and dance.

The developing child needs to have the right opportunity to move at the right time. The urge to crawl, stand up, climb, explore, feel and discover seems to arise spontaneously. Babies and toddlers need the time and space in which to practise.

The Principles

The Medau movement is a formalized but natural system, which has developed from the body structure and does not impose any distortion or rigidity. It is strong, flowing, rhythmical and dynamic. There are no jerky repetitious exercises and no overstretching. The main aim is to produce a lithe strong body totally at ease and in harmony with itself.

Heinrich Medau was a teacher of music and physical education who founded his own teacher training college in Berlin in 1929. He was an enthusiastic and expert exponent of the new mode of rhythmic movement, which was gradually replacing the old forms of rigid army-style exercise.

The Medau movement was part of an enthusiasm for going 'back to nature', along with the less strict and rigid approach to education pursued by teachers such as Steiner, Pestalozzi and Montessori. In the dance world, Isadora Duncan, with her 'free dance to natural rhythms', was another great influence.

Heinrich Medau had taught and studied children's movement, observing that it was effortless, economical, elastic and 'continuous through the body'. He called it 'natural whole body movement'. In working with children he aimed to preserve this natural talent, seeking to provide time and a safe, stimulating environment where natural movement play patterns could emerge, develop and be built on in the children's own time.

As a music teacher, Medau was very aware of small children's instinctive responses to and enjoyment of rhythm. He believed that 'Rhythm is the key to correct movement.' The human response to rhythm is one of the world's great mysteries. It seems to unlock the energy in the body, stimulating, motivating, supporting, and harmonizing movement.

Medau's work has been developed in many fields of physical education all over the world. As well as being in use with mother and toddler groups, and in ante- and postnatal classes, the Medau movement has also been adapted for work with the elderly, special needs groups, physiotherapy and remedial classes, stage movement classes, fitness and sport training courses, and dance. It is also an element in the healing therapies.

The Class

A class for toddlers and babies based on Medau's principles will always include the mother or minder and about 15 to 20 babies. There is a warm, easy atmosphere with a feeling of friendliness and approval for all. It is non-competitive, with no achievement grid to live up to, and the individual needs of the children are paramount.

The under threes work with an adult or older child. They are still, at this stage, very top-heavy and therefore apt to fall easily. No toddler should be allowed to change levels without supervision.

Ideas for what the children do are suggested, but never forced. There is always time to take things at their own pace and, in a good class, every suggestion as to how things should best be done is bound to be welcomed and properly explored.

The teaching is improvized on movement themes, in a way which is manageable and right for each age group. The teacher leads the group, joining in, demonstrating and generally setting the tone and pace.

Light hand apparatus, such as balls, hoops, bean bags, cushions and special soft toys, are used to stimulate and encourage the children and are an integral part of movement play. Sometimes gym apparatus, such as benches, boxes, small trampolines and a tunnel of chairs, is used to build a 'track'.

Social skills – politeness, waiting your turn, helpfulness and being part of the group, 'building', playing together, tidying away, greetings, thankyous and goodbyes – all these achievements are considered important. Each child is greeted and named.

Children are encouraged to work either barefoot, or wearing light plimsolls rather than cumbersome trainers. Surplus clothes are arranged tidily and put out of the way.

Classes for Two to Three Year Olds
These last approximately forty minutes and are improvised. The music is taped, not continuous, and is always carefully suited to a particular movement theme.

1 Space Work The children start exploring the space: they walk about the room or are carried. Then they form a circle, move in (let's make a tiny circle) and move out. Thereafter they might play at: run and touch the wall; let's all run to that corner; let's all sit on the floor and make a huddle. Other games include: Can you make a line? Shall we do 'Follow-my-leader'? Who's got some good ideas for an animal we can be? A camel? An elephant? Let's creep like a snake along the floor.

Below. *'I'm a dinosaur dragging my legs. Shall we be tiny mice with noses near the floor? Come close – let's make a mouse huddle together'* (see inset).

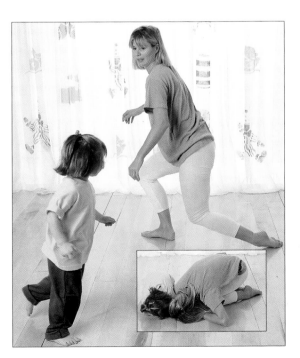

2 Warming Up and Letting Off Steam There's a general feeling of energy and fun as the children practise several exercises: marching steps, stamping, clapping and punching the air, tiptoes, running and skipping, gallops, rolling, and sideways gallops.

Below. *'Let's warm our legs, picking up one then the other, and rock as high as we can. Make a fist* (bottom) *and hit the air – pow! – that gets us warm.'*

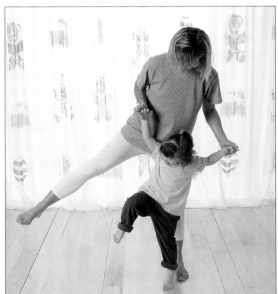

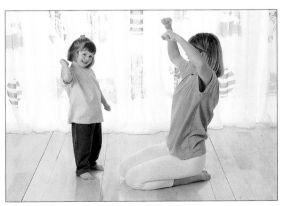

3 Stretching This game involves you asking: can you make a star? touch the ceiling? point east and west (horizontal stretch)? make your legs long? stretch your mouth open? stretch your fingers? Sometimes the child sits on the minder's lap and they both stretch out their arms and legs together.

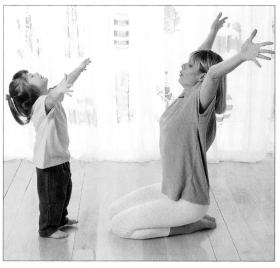

Above. *'Reach for the sky; stretch upwards. Can you touch the ceiling? Open your hands, wiggle your fingertips. Look up – can you see the stars?'*

Left. *'Hold my hands so you can balance and not fall over. Stretch out each leg as far as you can.'*

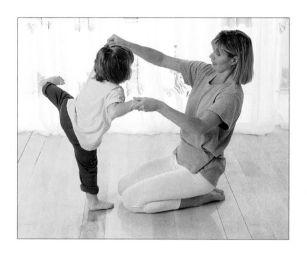

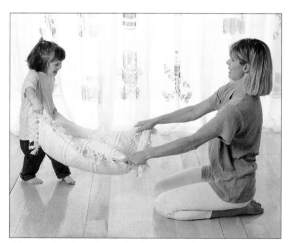

Above. *'Let's pick up this heavy cushion. We'd better try together. You hold one end while I take the other; now let's both heave. Lift your side higher than mine; now my end goes up. Shall we swing it from side to side – rock it – gently? Feel how heavy it is!'*

4 Strength Work This is often practised using a cushion or soft ball. The children play a variety of games: hug and squeeze the cushion tightly; tug it away from me; lift the cushion up; punch it; and carry it on your head – see how heavy it is!

A towel is also useful for this kind of play. It can be deployed in a tug of war, or in the game of rocking back and forth while you pull in opposite directions.

Still holding on to facing ends of the towel, you can flap it vigorously up and down to make a pretend breeze: 'You try it – see if you can cool me down.' This is a good way of showing your child how to use her whole back more strongly. With the towel's ends twisted up, she can also enjoy the game of 'Let's both thump it hard at the ground: thwack! thwack!'

5 Mobility This takes the form of questions combined with movement. The children are asked: who can show me a joint? your elbow – your knees, ankles and shoulders – how do they move? Nod your head – yes, yes. Shake it – no, no, no. Wiggle your fingers – now wriggle your toes.

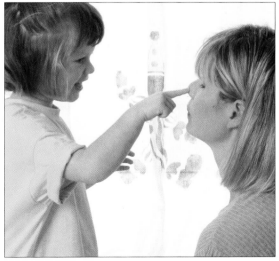

Above. *Your child will not find what parts she can move until she knows where everything is. Start very simply by asking, 'Show me your nose, hair, eyes, thumb. Where's my nose?' You can quickly progress to more difficult ideas, including combinations – 'Put your elbow on your knee.' Make it fun and keep it very light-hearted.*

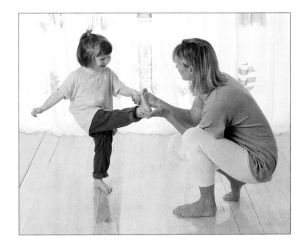

Above. *Explain to her, 'This is your ankle joint. It makes you move your foot. See how you can wave it. Point your toes up and down, then sideways. Can you make your foot go round and round? That's called rotating. Hold my hand and don't fall over.'*

Right. *Ask your child to lie on her back and see if she can catch her toes. Tell her, 'That moves your hip joint. See, your hands can make your legs go up and down.'*

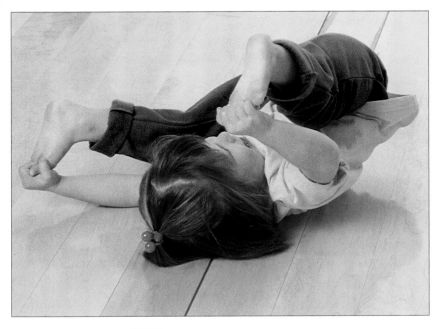

Right. *The time-honoured game of 'Round and round the garden like a teddy bear — one step, two steps, tickle you under there' — brings gleeful anticipation of being tickled.*

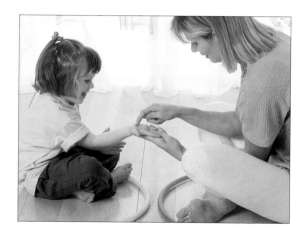

6 Group Work Togetherness Sometimes the children sing, or pass round a shared soft toy: we haven't seen our rabbit/teddy for ages — here he comes — shall we clap and cheer?

There are endless action rhymes to choose from. Children love rituals and follow the same songs and rhymes with increasing pleasure. These offer a bonding process of shared experience and fun.

7 Coordination and Agility Often a track is built for everyone to climb, balance and crawl along, running, jumping, creeping, and combining the movements in a sequence. A 'tunnel', cushions, small trampoline, large cushions, bench or chairs can be set out in a sequence. The children usually tackle this with excitement, finding it requires strength, concentration and agility. Much praise is given for any new skill.

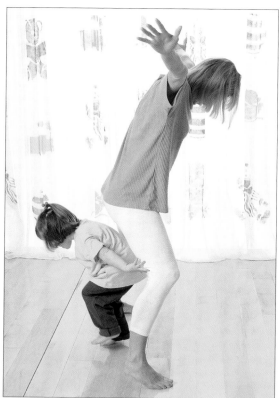

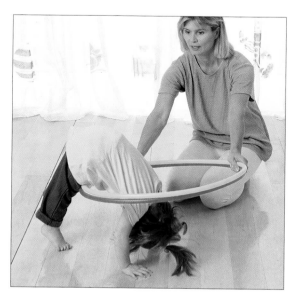

Above and left. *Encourage practising the skill of getting through a space. Going through a grown-up's legs calls for judging one's pace while tucking under. Head first through a hoop* (see left) *requires balance and concentration.*

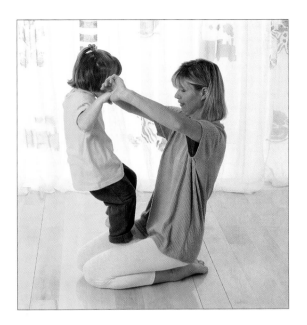

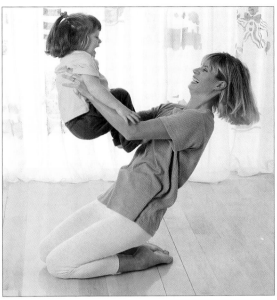

8 Goodbyes At the end of the session children and minders hold hands in a circle, say thank you to the group leaders, and turn to wave to themselves in the mirror.

Above. *Balancing on someone else demands sensitivity and timing. Ask 'Can you stand on my thighs?'* (left). *Then suggest 'See if you can walk up my tummy,' supporting her under the arms* (right).

At Home

Having observed that all living creatures, especially young ones, need to move as part of their development, it can be shocking to discover how many hours every day most babies are confined with no special safe place to play. They spend hours in car seats, buggies, and highchairs, being carried or wheeled round the supermarket or watching television. Time to explore, experiment and play is at a premium. They have always to fit in with the rest of the family, trying to keep up or slow down. Nothing makes an energetic toddler more frustrated and furious.

• Try to find time every day when you can move and play together, giving your undivided attention (no telephone calls) and allowing time for your child to choose and suggest ideas.

• Find a safe space where your baby is free to move about. Be very aware that houses are not safe and toddlers have to learn about stairs, chairs, slippery baths, and hot teapots, for example. They need time to recognize dangers and become aware and confident.

• Have a good working knowledge of nature's development plan. That dreamy baby asleep in her car seat may become a tough, restless two year old who wants to climb and kick and run about. Be sure to make time on journeys and every day for enough movement.

• Encourage everyone in the household to play, dance, romp and move with the baby. Everybody's health and good spirits will improve enormously, and your delighted child will love it.

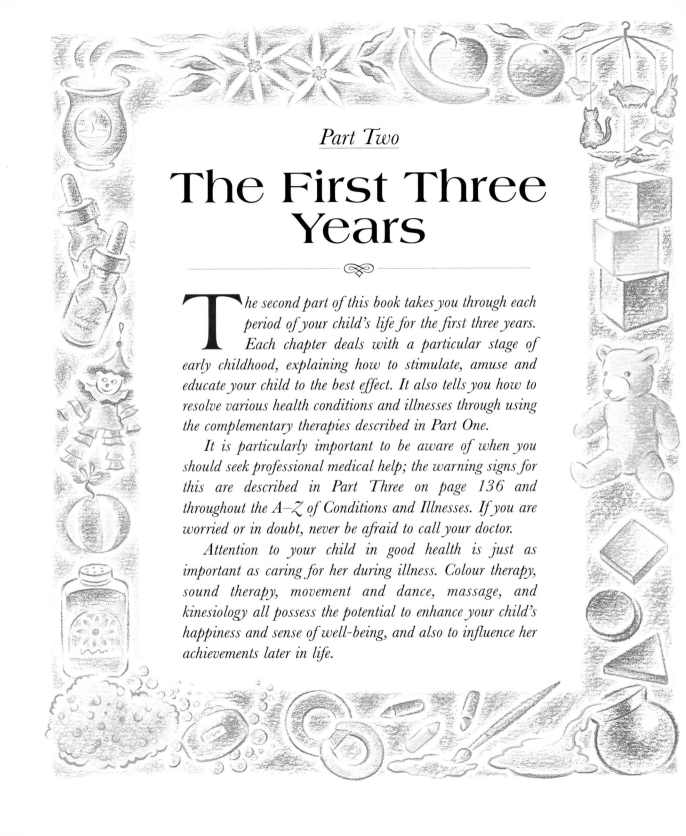

Part Two

The First Three Years

❧

The second part of this book takes you through each period of your child's life for the first three years. Each chapter deals with a particular stage of early childhood, explaining how to stimulate, amuse and educate your child to the best effect. It also tells you how to resolve various health conditions and illnesses through using the complementary therapies described in Part One.

It is particularly important to be aware of when you should seek professional medical help; the warning signs for this are described in Part Three on page 136 and throughout the A–Z of Conditions and Illnesses. If you are worried or in doubt, never be afraid to call your doctor.

Attention to your child in good health is just as important as caring for her during illness. Colour therapy, sound therapy, movement and dance, massage, and kinesiology all possess the potential to enhance your child's happiness and sense of well-being, and also to influence her achievements later in life.

CHAPTER ONE

Your Newborn Baby

As you take your baby to your breast in the first minute of new life, you will probably experience a turmoil of emotions and sensations. It may be that you find yourself simultaneously full of pleasure and weariness, of ecstasy and curiosity, and of relief.

Your baby will look at you, studying your face and taking in the smell of you. Right from the beginning of this, the first week of life, you, with your partner, are everything to this newborn person: her warmth, shelter, comfort and security. It will take time for you all to be completely bonded, but this will come. Some parents say that they fell in love with their baby the second they saw her, but this is not always the case. These first few minutes are of inestimable value to you and your partner and your baby, so do savour them before the midwife or other carer carries out the various routine checks.

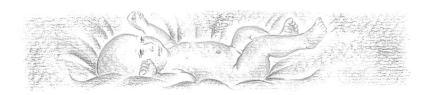

First Moments in the World

If you have given birth in a hospital your temperature will be taken and your pulse and blood pressure measured. Your baby will be weighed, measured in length and in head circumference, footprinted and given a name band. The baby's condition is then assessed according to the Apgar score (*shown below*).

Testing according to this score may be repeated after five minutes. Five things are checked as an indication of the baby's general health, and points awarded from 0 to 2 for each of the five factors. The infant that scores 10 will be in good general health. The signs are: respiratory effort (breathing); pulse rate; pallor (colour); muscular tone; and response to stimuli (reflexes).

Newborn babies often don't look completely beautiful, except perhaps to their parents, until a few days after their birth. By then the minor bumps and wrinkles caused by the journey down the birth canal have smoothed out. So don't be surprised if your baby has little bruises, the odd spot or rash and, possibly, enlarged breasts and genitals (these are caused by hormonal fluctuations which settle soon after birth). The umbilical cord will be clamped and cut when it has stopped pulsating after the birth and the clamped stump at the baby's navel left to drop off of its own accord.

The baby will be given the Guthrie test for phenylketonuria and hypothyroidism. These are diseases which, if untreated, cause mental impairment. They are simply detected by taking a small blood sample from the baby and analysing it. If the diseases are found to be present, the baby can be treated with complete success. If the mother has tuberculosis, or is likely to have been exposed to TB, her baby will be offered a BCG vaccination (bacille Calmette-Guérin, named after the doctors who formulated it) shortly after delivery. BCG may also be offered to parents who are likely to have visitors or relatives from parts of the world where tuberculosis is still prevalent; likewise if the family plan to visit such countries in the first few years of the baby's life.

From a developmental point of view, the newborn baby is still in a foetal stage, a state of

Apgar Score			
Sign	**Responses**		
Respiratory effort	None	Weak cry, slow breathing	Good strong cry
Pulse	None	Slow, under 100 beats per minute	Fast (over 100 per minute)
Skin colour	Blue and very pale	Blue and no pallor	All pink
Muscular tone	Limp	Some flexing of fingers and toes	Active, fingers and toes flexing well
Response to stimuli (reflex irritability)	No response	Grimace	Cry
Score	O	1	2

total dependence, unlike that of most other mammals' young. She needs to be in close bodily contact with her mother during the first months of life. Your baby should never be isolated in a separate room, nor left alone for long periods. Lay her on your body and let her feel the rhythm of your breath and your heartbeat. Look into her eyes and exchange feelings. Introduce colours, harmonious sounds, soothing balanced music, fragrances and touch, letting your fingers explore. And, most importantly, allow the presence of quietness. Sway or rock your baby to sleep.

Your baby is very receptive to smell. If she is born into an environment perfumed with essential oils, her brain may well register the aroma. Research has shown, too, that babies can smell their way to the breast at birth. While you are both still in the delivery room, put her to your breast, and ask the midwife if you can share some quiet moments alone.

Breast-feeding Routines

This is a time for establishing routines of feeding and hygiene which make life more agreeable in the long term for both parents and baby. Once breast-feeding is successfully established, do you feed on demand or do you keep to a simple timetable?

Some midwives, experienced in natural childbirth and rearing, recommend a pattern of only four or five feeds a day at regular intervals as being the best way to achieve contented children and parental peace. At other times the baby should be comforted when necessary but not breast-fed. With the last feed at around 10 pm, the baby will usually sleep through to about 6 am and will tend to have less colic or digestive discomfort if she is not constantly taking irregular feeds.

To help this work well, it is important for you to feed the baby, especially the last feed at around 10 pm, in quiet surroundings. Try to make sure that you are free of any distractions, intrusions, or interruptions such as television or the telephone.

Difficulties with breast-feeding such as a low milk supply, mastitis or cracked nipples can all be alleviated by professional homoeopathic attention. Ring your homoeopath, who will help you with advice on finding the most appropriate remedy.

The Herbal Options

Use	Herbs (in combination or alone)	Method
To bathe your newborn baby (calming and cleansing)	Lavender, chamomile, rosemary, limeflowers, lemon balm, or rose petals	Add infusions to bath water
To clean the eyes and face, and the nappy area	Lavender, marigold, chamomile, rosewater	Antiseptic infusions
To help parents and baby recover	Rescue Remedy, walnut, Star of Bethlehem	As Bach flower remedies
To restore the mother after the birth	Cloves, ginger and cinnamon with raspberry leaves, or Chinese angelica	Decoction
To enhance breast-feeding, production of breast milk	Holy thistle, raspberry leaves, fennel, dill, goat's rue, borage, and nettles, vervain, cinnamon, chaste tree	As a tea

Recovering Your Strength

To encourage restful sleep following labour, and to help allay the tensions brought on by excitement and hormonal fluctuations: sprinkle 1–2 drops of essential oil such as neroli, rose, ylang ylang or lavender on a tissue and inhale deeply. Keep the tissue beside you while you rest.

After months of waiting and hoping, the emotional upheaval of giving birth will have been enormous. This may be even more so if labour has been physically gruelling, and lasted several hours.

Relieving Discomfort

To help prevent and heal infection and relieve soreness from stitches or bruising: to a warm bath add 2 drops of lavender and 2 drops of cypress, swish the water to mix these essential oils, and relax for 10 minutes.

Alternatively, use a compress (*see page 14*), adding 2 drops each of lavender and cypress to 300ml cold water. Use a disposable cloth or sterile maternity pad to hold the compress against the perineum. For a very sore perineal area or haemorrhoids, wrap a lavender- or cypress-soaked cloth around crushed ice (or a small pack of frozen peas) and apply to the affected area.

To relieve bruising after the birth take a dose of Arnica 200; for soreness, a dose of Calendula 200. Both will speed up the healing of the uterus and perineum. If you experience a post-partum fever, call your homoeopath immediately for effective treatment.

The Homoeopathic Options

Condition	Remedy	How to Use
Sore and bruised perineum	Arnica 200 and Calendula 200	Should be given after delivery. Bathing the perineum in a dilution of Hypercal tincture is also beneficial.
Difficulty in breast-feeding due to prolonged jaundice in the newborn (very common problem at this age)	Chelidonium 30	Two-hourly for a day
Colicky, bad-tempered babies, colic worse from 4 to 8 pm	Lycopodium 30	For instructions on dosage (*see page 33*)
Difficulties in breast-feeding (can lead to problems such as mastitis)	Bryonia, Phytolacca, Conium, Belladonna, or other remedies can be prescribed effectively by a homoeopath	For instructions on dosage (*see page 33*)
Dwindling breast milk	The appropriate remedy to increase milk can be prescribed by your homoeopath	Your homoeopath will advise you on dosage
Cracked nipples	Castor equii 30	For instructions on dosage (*see page 33*)
Parental fatigue; dizziness and disorientation, often due to lack of sleep	Cocculus 30	For instructions on dosage (*see page 33*)

Aromatic Solutions
Stretch Marks

These are thin pink or red lines caused by weakening of underlying fibres in the skin. The breasts will be susceptible to stretch marks because of their fluctuating size. Wear a good-fitting bra night and day. To help the breasts to retain elasticity and suppleness, keep them well nourished by making up a bottle of the following oil: to 80ml almond or grapeseed oil add essential oil in the form of 7 drops of lavender and 5 drops of tangerine or mandarin. Massage a small amount of the oil over the breasts up to the collar bone and around the tops of arms daily. The same oil can be used to massage abdomen, thighs, hips and bottom (until your pre-baby weight is regained, these areas will still be prone to stretch marks). Breast-feeding helps considerably in preventing stretch marks on the breast.

Engorged Breasts

This condition usually occurs during the first week. The breasts become lumpy and/or swollen and painful and the baby may find it difficult to feed. To help relieve pressure and swelling, make a compress as follows. To 300ml either hot (for pressure) or cold (for swelling) water, add essential oils: 2 drops of geranium and 2 drops of lavender. Soak a cloth and hold against the breast. Try and express some milk to relieve the fullness.

You can add 2 drops of lavender and 2 drops of geranium to a hot bath. Gently massage your breasts under the water.

Use 2 drops of geranium to 10ml almond oil to massage your breasts (avoid the nipple area) after feeding the baby. This will help prevent congestion occurring. Before giving your baby the next feed, wipe the skin around your nipple in case any oil remains.

Resting

Mother, as well as baby, will need plenty of rest in these early weeks. Try and plan to have a siesta yourself in the middle of the day when you can lie flat and allow the pressure on over-stretched pelvic tissues to be relieved. Place two pillows under your legs to raise them above the level of the abdomen. This helps the veins of the legs to drain.

Your diet should be light and nutritious with no tea, coffee, alcohol, or refined foods. Remember that everything you eat and drink while breast-feeding is passed to your baby.

This very early stage of babyhood passes so quickly; relish it while it lasts, and sleep and relax as much as you wish.

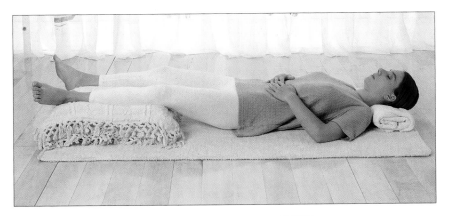

Left. *The ideal position for relaxing. Choose any firm, even surface, such as your bed or a folded rug on the floor. Rest for twenty or thirty minutes if possible with the fingers lightly touching across your middle, and legs and feet quite loose. Support your neck with a small pillow or rolled-up towel.*

The Power of Touch

During birth the baby has received her first massage as she is squeezed, stroked and stretched on her way down the birth canal into the outside world.

From a curled up position in a cramped space your baby is thrust, or pulled, or lifted, into a world without boundaries where she has as yet no idea of the space she occupies. As she reaches out she can no longer touch the sides of her environment. This is a very puzzling and challenging time.

More and more people are becoming aware of the sort of welcome a baby needs most. While the baby lies naked on the mother's bare belly, bonding already begins. The mother will instinctively reach out to touch her even though the baby may look a bit odd: wrinkled, bloody and covered in vernix, a greasy substance thought to protect the baby's skin and insulate against heat loss.

The loving touch begins as mother strokes her baby's back and touches the head, exploring the little body.

Close contact continuously during the first week is the best way to establish a good relationship with the child. Many mothers spend much of that early time just gazing at their newborn. Close physical contact can convey the sheer joy of motherhood and ensure that the baby is constantly reassured and made secure and content.

Handling Your Baby

Babies let you know what they like and protest loudly if things don't suit them exactly. They are the best guide for what they prefer and what is good for them.

Firm Hands

Being much more physically tough than one might imagine, babies like a sure touch. Delicate 'feather' fingers are out – the baby feels insecure.

Squeeze your hands into a fist and rub them together, warming the palms and feeling the energy you've stimulated. Pick up, change,

Right. *Lying down with your baby on your tummy can be very relaxing for both of you. You become more aware of your own breathing, and its rhythm also soothes the baby. Being physically so close to you, she can feel your heartbeat, which perhaps reminds her of the months she spent in the womb. Whether through clothes or not, use a firm, calming hand to stroke her down the length of the spine.*

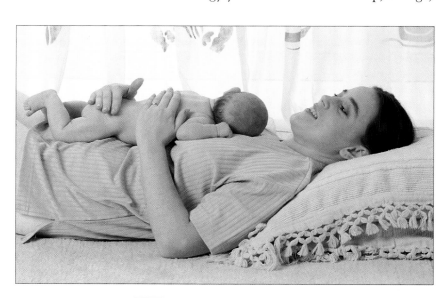

dress or bath the baby, remembering that she is likely to be calmed by the feel of firm hands.

Tense Touch

Since the way in which we feel physically will affect our mental and emotional outlook, then releasing muscular tension through the use of the Alexander technique will help us to be calmer and generally happier in our day-to-day lives. Your newborn baby will sense this improvement and she will often be more content as a result. It is often easy for someone who is not emotionally involved with a family to see a nervous or anxious mother transferring her own tension to her infant. Even the actual birth may be less stressful if the people in attendance and the surroundings are harmonious and calm – midwives can often tell in advance what sort of birth the mother will have, simply by how calm she is.

If either the mother or child have experienced trauma during the birth, the Alexander technique can help to reduce any muscular tension. By putting into practice the lessons you have learned from your practitioner, you may be able to treat this tension even years after the birth. The birth of your child is a miraculous occasion, and the more conscious and aware you are during those first few days the more you will enjoy the whole experience, thus giving your child the best possible start in life. Having Alexander lessons and being more 'conscious' and more aware of your body, can really help you to savour those precious moments when you meet the one who is to become so important in your life.

Baby Gym

Unless the birth has been difficult and the baby distressed and needing to be quiet, you cannot start to move, rock, cuddle and sing soon enough. Life in the womb is full of sound, movement, rhythms, change of pressure and posture and this should be allowed to continue. Thus playtime begins at once. Sitting up in bed, wrap or bundle your baby lightly, hold her closely and rock gently forwards and backwards. Sing or hum if you like. Remember all those old nursery rhymes such as 'Hush-a-bye-baby'. Your baby will love the sound of your soft singing.

The Cranio-sacral Check

In an ideal world, a cranio-sacral therapist would attend every birth (or all midwives would be trained in cranio-sacral therapy). With this advantage, it would be easier to relieve the mother's pain and tension; to provide a more comfortable and less traumatic birth for the baby; and, above all, to check the baby immediately after birth.

In the majority of cases a brief check-up is sufficient to ensure that the fundamental energy of the cranio-sacral system is strong and that there are no major distortions or compressions. A weak system might contribute to cot death. Severe distortions or compressions might cause brain damage or cerebral palsy, so it is important to remedy these problems at the earliest opportunity.

Assuming there is nothing severe, there is no further need for treatment in the first two weeks. A baby's cranium can be naturally distorted during its passage through the birth canal and may emerge in a strange shape. This is usually nothing to be alarmed about. It is part of nature's design that the head be soft and malleable so that it can squeeze through this narrow channel.

A cranio-sacral check-up is all the more important if the birth was difficult, if labour was prolonged, if the baby was under stress, if contractions stopped – particularly during the second stage – if the baby had been stuck at any time, if, while still in the womb, there was any unusual position (for example, with a hand up beside the head), if a lot of medication was given, or if forceps or a ventouse was used. If the baby seems reasonably happy and healthy then the system is best allowed to settle of its own accord for two weeks. After this a craniosacral check-up is recommended for all babies, even if the birth was easy and there have been no obvious symptoms.

Your Baby's Perception

Unlike the sense of sound, a baby's vision has been of little use to her while in the womb, but it has been proven that the foetus will react to light. In experiments where a bright light has been shone on to the uterus, the foetus has responded by moving abruptly away. It is not until the moment of birth however that a baby's vision starts to develop rapidly. This is mainly due to the sudden bombardment of stimuli. At first, sight is very poor, slightly out of focus and lacks definition. Focus is limited to objects less than a metre away. A newborn baby is able to see in colour – except that she is thought unable to see the colour blue. Research carried out on newborns has shown that they are attracted to and look for moving objects. A second visual preference is for very high-contrast objects such as those that are striped or chequered.

Your Baby's Aura

Colour is not absorbed into the body by the eyes alone but also through the skin. Each pore of a baby's skin can be likened to a microscopic eye, so that the colour of the clothes worn by a baby will also have an effect on it. Anything that is rubbed into the skin or placed on the skin will be absorbed into the body.

A newborn baby has a sensitive and delicate aura which is filled with very pale ethereal colours. It would therefore be inadvisable to dress such a young infant in bright, vibrant colours, because these could be detrimental to the child. One colour which is very beneficial is white. This contains all the colours, allowing the infant to absorb what she requires. Other favoured colours are pastel shades of blue, pink or yellow. Blue induces peace and tranquillity, and is therefore a good colour for a restless baby. Very pale pink is the colour of unconditional love, and can be very comforting to a newborn baby that has spent nine months cocooned in the warmth and safety of its mother's womb before being propelled into the strange and busy world. Yellow, apart from being a bright sunny colour, works with the intellect and can be advantageous for stimulating the infant's rapidly developing brain.

CHAPTER TWO

Getting to Know You

By now, at the end of the first week of your new baby's life, you will have begun to get to know each other a little. You will soon be able to distinguish the different sorts of cries your baby will make – of recognition, of pleasure, of cold, of hunger, of longing for company.

Bonding is all-important at this stage. Teachers of the Alexander technique recognize that the more 'present' and generally aware you are, the quicker this process will be. The technique can help you to enjoy your baby during these first three months of her life, by teaching you how to focus fully. Many mothers are pressurized into going back to work too early, which can be detrimental to both them and their child. This also goes against one of the principles of the Alexander technique, which is not to become too goal orientated. The mother needs to forget worldly ambitions and immerse herself in caring for her baby.

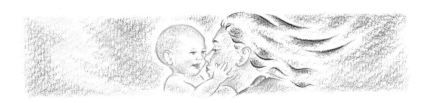

The Power of Touch

Of course you may worry as you realize that you are entirely responsible for this little bundle's welfare. The human newborn is the most helpless of creatures. But although your baby is tiny, and seemingly fragile, she needs touching with confidence. If the mother is nervous or afraid, this will be communicated to the baby. Before starting the following massage, go back to Part One and re-read the seven important Do's and Don'ts. Also take another look at the Positions for Massage section (*see pages 18 and 19*).

Massaging Your Baby

The aim of massage for your baby is communication through loving touch, to soothe and comfort or to stimulate and enliven. The pace and pressure of your massage will determine the result. Simply, if massage is given slowly and smoothly it will relax, if fast and brisk, it will stimulate.

Allow your hands to sense what your baby needs, and use your strokes to follow the contours of the little body. Often, closing your eyes allows you to 'see' more when massaging.

Right, inset. *Lay the baby on his back. Maintain eye contact while talking or singing to him. Warm the oil in your hands and place them on the front of your baby's chest. Use one hand if your baby is very small but touch or hold another part of him with your other hand.*

Right. *Glide your hands from the middle to the sides of the baby's chest. Use most pressure on the chest and the front of his shoulders, and less as you return your hands under each side of the ribcage. Feel their pressure relaxing the muscles, widening the shoulders and so aiding your baby's breathing. Repeat these movements three or four times.*

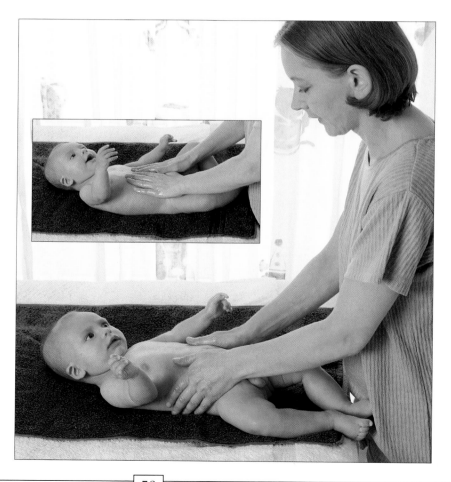

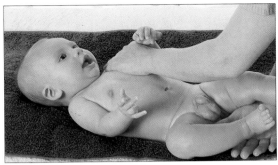

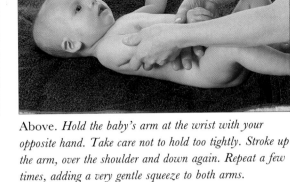

Above. *Circle back to the middle of the chest. Try not to lose contact with the baby's skin. Glide each hand in turn to the opposite shoulder, then over and back to the centre of his chest. Repeat two or three times.*

Above. *Hold the baby's arm at the wrist with your opposite hand. Take care not to hold too tightly. Stroke up the arm, over the shoulder and down again. Repeat a few times, adding a very gentle squeeze to both arms.*

Left. *Massage the belly down towards the groin, one hand following the other repeatedly in an almost circular action. Do not massage the umbilicus if it is still healing.*

Below left. *Stroke down the leg towards the foot. Again, exert a gentle squeeze along the way.*

Below right. *Use your thumb to circle into the sole of the foot. Gently press and stretch each toe in turn (bottom). Finish one leg before starting on the other.*

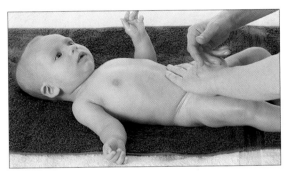

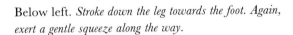

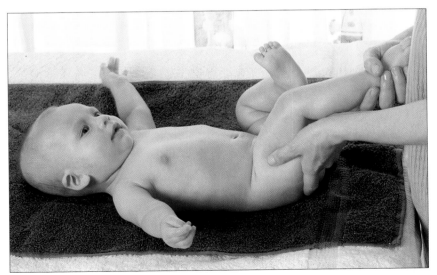

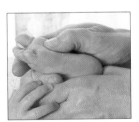

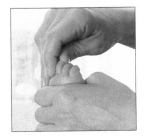

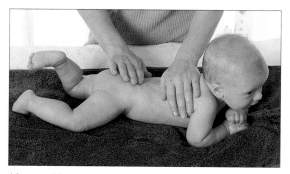 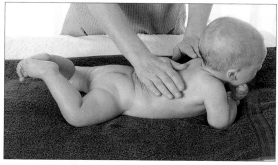

Above. *Turn the baby over. The amount of oil used should be enough to allow your hands to glide easily over your baby's skin but not so much that he is difficult to handle. Start by rubbing your hands back and forth across the baby's back, moving them slowly up and down.*

Above. *Using one hand, stroke firmly down from the neck to the bottom of the spine. While you do so, he will often lift his head, making the muscles feel quite taut. Notice the difference when he rests his head and the muscles relax. Repeat three or four times.*

Right. *Make small circles over the baby's back with your fingers. Feel the bones of the spinal column, placing your fingertips close beside each vertebra. Starting from the neck, work down one side of the spine; then go back to the neck and repeat the same movements down the other side.*

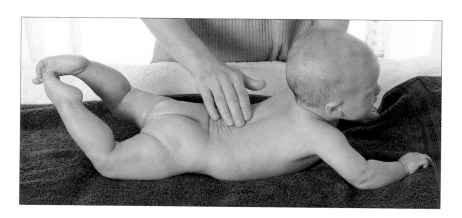

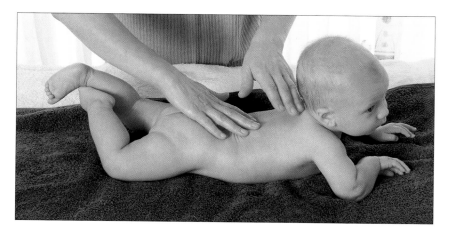

Left. *Finish with light finger-strokes to signal the last stage of the massage. Repeat, with both hands getting lighter each time. In the end you will find that you are barely touching the skin. Cover your baby immediately you have finished, preferably wrapping him in a warm towel, and give him a great big cuddle.*

Aromatic Massage

Babies thrive on massage, for it strengthens the bonding process and helps to develop a special closeness and communication between parent and child. The baby feels secure; she also learns her first lessons on how to receive and give pleasure.

When massaged regularly, babies feed and sleep well, and are less likely to be troubled with colic and constipation.

By incorporating gentle essential oils into the massage routine, you will increase its benefits in several ways.

You will encourage associations between pleasing aromas and happy relaxed times. In addition, you will be keeping your baby contented and happy, and soothing away any

When Massaging Don't...

- *Don't attempt a massage when hurried or when the baby is fretful.*

- *Don't spend longer than five minutes on each massage while your baby is younger than eight weeks. Ten minutes is the maximum for an older baby.*

- *Don't massage your baby's hands with oil as this may then be transferred to the mouth or eyes. Also avoid the face, as the oil could seep into the eyes.*

- *Don't use clear mineral-based baby oils as the base carrier oil. Use, instead, almond oil or a mix of almond and jojoba oil in which to dilute and mix the essential oil of your choice.*

Your Baby's Aromatic Environment

Where to Use	Which Essential Oil	How to Use
Nappy bucket for pre-wash	Tea tree	6 drops in bucket soak
Washing machine – nappies	Lavender	4 drops in final rinse compartment
Sink, for washing nappies	Lavender	2 drops in final rinse by hand
Baby's clothes wash – by machine	Roman chamomile, lavender or neroli	4 drops in final rinse compartment
Tumble dryer – with clothes	Lavender, geranium, bergamot, sandalwood, rosemary or ylang ylang	4–8 drops on small piece of fabric (a single old sock is ideal)
Airing cupboard	Neroli, petitgrain, geranium or lavender	2–3 drops on cotton wool balls or on padded coathanger
Wiping down surfaces (in kitchen, on high chair, in bathroom)	Lemon, bergamot, lavender, eucalyptus or tea tree	4–6 drops in solution of 300ml water
Any room to remove smells and help prevent spread of germs	Bergamot, eucalyptus, tea tree, lavender or geranium	Fill sprayer with 300ml water and 6 drops chosen oil and spray oil mist
Any room to bring calming atmosphere	Ylang ylang, mandarin or lavender	Fill sprayer with 300ml water and 6 drops chosen oil and spray oil mist

aches and pains. Her skin will be clean and sweet smelling; it will also be free from the bacteria that cause nappy rash; moreover you will be helping to boost your baby's general immunity to disease.

As well as smelling deliciously fragrant, essential oils are natural disinfectants and antiseptics, being both anti-bacterial and anti-viral in their effect.

They also have an advantage over commercial kinds of air-fresheners, which appear to banish odours merely by covering them up. By contrast, vaporized essential oils are able to cut right through bad smells, in the course of rapidly disinfecting and cleaning the air.

Essential Oils for Baby Massage

When massaging your baby, try oils such as Roman chamomile, rose, lavender, tangerine, neroli. Try any of the following combinations:

• *to 50ml almond oil, or 30ml almond oil and 20ml jojoba oil mixed, add 1 drop of Roman chamomile, rose, lavender or neroli;*

• *to 100ml almond oil, or 80ml almond oil and 20ml jojoba oil mixed, add 1 drop of chamomile and 1 drop of rose mixed, or 1 drop of lavender oil and 1 drop of neroli.*

Feeding Your Baby

The Alexander technique enables you to find a comfortable position for breastfeeding, whether lying or sitting. Your baby may be feeding for many hours a day, and sitting in awkward positions can produce aches and pains both in you and the baby. Through the technique's principles you can prevent or alleviate many of these discomforts and lessen the baby's likelihood of colic. It can also improve self-esteem and give you more confidence as a mother which, in turn, will help you

Right. *You may find yourself in one position for long periods while feeding your baby. If this position is uncomfortable it may produce unnecessary tension and can cause backache or neckache.*

Far right. *Using cushions under your baby's head and under your foot can help prevent the problems of tension caused by bad posture.*

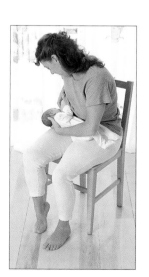

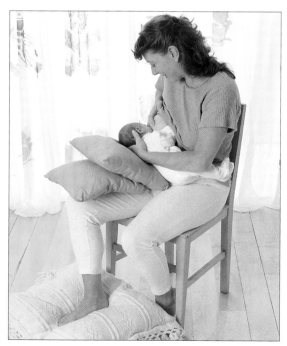

to persevere with breast-feeding when the process seems difficult. With breast-feeding proceeding smoothly, you will also not be in a hurry to wean your child. Suckling as soon as possible after birth is important to stimulate milk production and establish feeding.

Breast-feeding can sometimes take a while to establish. It is not unusual to take as long as a month for it to become a comfortable experience for both mother and baby. The nipples will often be sore and cracked. The breasts may engorge and feel hot and hard.

Expression may be necessary. Not all women want to breast-feed. Some feel the breasts to be part of their sexual attraction and they may resent the intense commitment that this method of feeding requires.

Nonetheless, breast-feeding can allow you to communicate and bond deeply with your baby. In the middle of the night, it feels as though there is just you and your baby, together making a connection to the natural order. There is no more intimate or exclusive way of building on your relationship.

Parental Fatigue

Massage

In Indian villages, mothers are massaged immediately after giving birth. There is no better way of getting back in touch with your body and beginning the recovery process. Tired, aching and sore, elated, nervous and overwhelmed, you can find that massage helps restore your equilibrium and contributes to more positive, confident feelings. Have your partner massage you, perhaps with aromatic oils. Use 5 drops of essential oil to 10ml of any carrier oil, for a body massage.

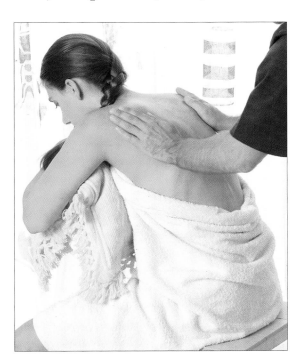

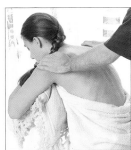

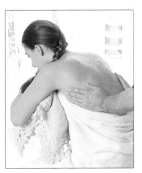

Left. *Shoulder Massage. Warm the oil in your hands. Start low on either side of the spine and glide the hands upwards* (far left). *Follow the spine and spread the stroke out to the top of the arms. Release the pressure* (top left) *and relax your hands as you bring them lightly back to the starting position. Repeat this stroke several times so that you cover the exposed area. Start some strokes with hands further apart* (bottom left) *and widen them by degrees. Check the pressure with your partner.*

Essential Oils

Essential oils to reduce parental fatigue can be either relaxing or revivifying.

• *Calming and relaxing oils to use at bedtime: mandarin, ylang ylang, rose, lavender, neroli, jasmine, Roman chamomile.*
• *Reviving and uplifting oils: geranium, rosemary, bergamot, lemon.*
• *Add 4–6 drops of any of the essential oils listed above to your bath.*
• *Foot massage: 5 drops of any of the above oils to 10ml of any carrier oil.*

Visualization

Lastly, keep 10–15 minutes for yourself, to perform this relaxing visualization technique in an aromatic atmosphere.

Place 1–2 drops of any of the following essential oils on a tissue and slowly inhale for a calming effect: petitgrain, geranium, mandarin, bergamot, ylang ylang, lavender. At the same time that you inhale, close your eyes and tune into your breathing.

Let your thoughts slowly drift away and imagine instead that you are walking, very slowly, along a tropical beach. The beach is deserted. You have all the time in the world. No one wants you to do anything for them. The white sand is warm beneath your bare feet and the sun is gently warming your shoulders. You lie on the sand and relax, feeling warm and contented. Meanwhile, you can hear the gentle rhythmic lapping of the waves on the shore and your breathing calms down further in association with the lapping of the water. Let go of your body as you relax, and allow all your former tensions to float away.

When you feel ready, open your eyes slowly ... and slowly come to. You will feel refreshed.

Baby Blues

Aromatic oils, especially rose, will comfort you and chase away the melancholy feelings that are so common after giving birth. Brought on by hormonal changes after birth, these emotions usually pass quite swiftly, but in the mean time they bring a sense of depression that can be very distressing for both mother and partner. They are most likely to occur around the third to fifth day after the delivery. You may just find yourself very tearful for no apparent reason. This should only last a couple of days. If it persists, see your doctor. Post-natal depression needs taking seriously.

Choose any of the following essential oils, or mix two or three of them together: rose, neroli, ylang ylang or bergamot. Add 4–5 drops to your bath or use the oils in a carrier oil to massage your hands and feet. Alternatively, put 1–2 drops on a tissue and slowly inhale.

Skin Care

Hormonal and emotional upsets can affect the condition of your skin, making it excessively dry, oily, or prone to spots. Incorporating essential oils into a simple regime of regular skin-care can have a two-fold effect. Firstly, this can improve the texture and condition of the skin; in addition it will encourage the formation of healthy new cells.

The fragrance will also have a calming effect, lifting your mood and helping you feel more cheerful and relaxed.

Jojoba facial oil will nourish and improve skin tone and help you to feel relaxed. To 10ml jojoba oil stir in 2 drops of any of these essential oils: rose, sandalwood, neroli, jasmine, Roman chamomile. Use a little of the mixed formula to massage your face or hands. Rub some into your wrists and use as a perfume to inhale when you feel tense.

Your Baby's Perception

Newborn babies have a very simple mental template of the human face and will search out and stare at human faces during their first two months of life. This means that they will be attracted to the people who care for them during their early life, namely their mother and father. When a baby is cradled in its mother's arms, it is at the perfect distance to see her face. Babies are still unable to focus clearly on distant objects at this age.

Awareness of Shape and Colour

At four weeks of age, a baby will track a moving object and focus on where it rests. It is learning to locate things. After eight weeks, it starts to become interested in the shape and colour of objects.

At this age, a mobile hung over the cot will cause great interest. This could consist of six or seven different shapes, each in a different colour. The colours need to be pastel shades of blue, yellow, pink, turquoise, orange and violet. In one experiment, two- to three-month-old babies were placed on their backs with a complex mobile hanging above their heads. Each baby had one ankle attached to the mobile with a satin ribbon. When, by chance, the babies wriggled the attached foot, they discovered that they could make the mobile move. Once they had learnt this, they constantly jerked their foot in order to turn the mobile. This continued when their foot was untied. When the objects on the mobile were then changed to a different colour, each baby stopped moving its foot.

This indicates that a baby's memory is very dependent on details of the context in which an experience first occurred and that colour plays a large part in this experience. Up to the age of three months, a baby has difficulty in disengaging from an interesting toy. This is one reason why the toys surrounding the infant should be in pastel shades. Harsh colours could make their eyes tired. One way of moving their focus of attention is by creating a sound. This can be done with either a rattle or the voice. If using a rattle, try to find one that is in pastel colours.

In the same way that a baby will absorb the colour of the clothes she is wearing, she can also absorb the colour of her mother's clothes when being cradled by her. It would therefore be beneficial to wear blue when feeding or rocking the child to sleep. This colour will induce peace and relaxation in both mother and child. An infant can detect if her mother is angry or upset and will react accordingly.

If clothes are used as a filter for colour absorption, it is important that either white or nothing is worn beneath the colour garment. If the infant is wearing a blue outer garment, then it should wear white beneath it. If the mother wears blue when nursing the infant, then the infant should wear white or be naked. The reason for this is if two different colours are worn, daylight will pass through both colours and what the recipient receives is a mixture of these colours. For example, if a person wears a blue dress over yellow underwear, the colour that would be absorbed through the skin would be green.

Using Bates' Principles

Children's sight will develop normally if good conditions prevail. If, however, the child is subject to specific and unrelieved stresses, such as sibling rivalry, then development, including sight, can be impaired.

Sight is the primary sense through which our world is measured. Parents who practise the Bates method will be well placed to support the development and maintenance of good sight in their child. In fact, although there is not much to do, there is much to be aware of, since the act of seeing is totally passive. Thus, some of the method's help consists of not overdoing things, for example not over-stimulating the child or pushing her to read prematurely. Moreover, it is potentially harmful to the baby if the parents are preoccupied, irritable, driven to daydreams, stare or are bored. It is helpful to be interested, aware, attentive, accepting and to notice what is happening to your baby.

Children made to conform to restrictive codes of behaviour can grow up with their real needs and interests being neglected, rather like letting a garden become a wasteland. It is beneficial, however, to arrange clear and sensible boundaries, within which the child can feel free and at ease rather than constrained.

Enhancing Your Baby's Sight
The following Bates method procedures can be usefully applied to the first stages of life.
• Give your baby your full attention whenever you can.
• Give plenty of cuddles and hugs.
• Look deeply into your baby's eyes, exchanging wordless feeling. This open look doesn't last very long in infancy.

• Gently, with two fingers, run an infinity sign, '∞', round the bony orbits of the eyes, out along the eyebrows and in on the cheekbones.
• Ensure the baby's room is well lit.
• Change the position of the cot periodically, and avoid putting the cot against the wall. The baby needs to be approached from different sides otherwise she may get the impression of being one-sided.
• If bottle-feeding, remember to alternate the side of the baby against your body, to avoid pressure to only one eye.
• Speak to your baby from different parts of the room as you move around, to help her follow a moving object.
• Put her in as many different rooms and positions as possible during the day so that she sees as many different patterns of light and bright objects as possible.
• Hang a colourful mobile near the top of the cot to attract her interest.
• Give the baby a light rattle to play with, to help see, hear and feel at the same time.

Lastly, gradually increase your range of movement and experience to help the baby become alert and responsive. Play with your hands, making gestures. Yawn together: yawning stimulates energy flow, helps tear fluid to lubricate the eyes and assists the relaxation of jaw muscles. Gently trace infinity signs around the orbits of the baby's eyes once more.

Encouraging a Pattern for Sleep

As you get to know your baby and her responses to you and her surroundings, you will begin to know instinctively when you need to give a little more or less time on the breast. With a well-established feeding routine, you will be less likely to have disturbed nights, but if your baby does wake, you will need to comfort her for a while before putting her back to sleep. If she is really restless, try giving her a feed of warm water mixed with just a dab of honey in a bottle.

Where Your Baby Can Sleep
Use your own intuition and instincts rather than be told by other people how, or where, you should put your baby to sleep. In many

cultures, it is common to have the newborn in bed with the parents all night. The advantages of this practice are that the baby always has warmth and the mother does not have to get up in the night, which lessens the likelihood of her becoming over-tired and depressed.

The orthodox view is that it is unwise for a young baby to share a bed with her parents because of the risk of one or other of them rolling over and lying on her. Putting her to sleep in a cot positioned very close to the parental bed for the first three months of life could be a sensible compromise.

Coping With Crying

There are many different reasons for a baby continually crying.

It may be a sense of isolation (don't hesitate to take her into your bed with you) or it may be hunger, boredom, fear, indigestion or some other minor complaint, or an illness (*see Part Three for a list of conditions*).

The more tense the mother or father when the baby cries, the worse the situation often becomes. Alexander technique lessons can make the parents more relaxed and confident. This in turn will reassure the child.

Common Problems

In order to avoid indigestion, at the start of each breast-feed, once the baby has attached herself to the nipple, remove the nipple from her mouth after about five seconds and allow three or four seconds just to swallow what she has already sucked.

Repeat this once or twice, introducing longer intervals before withdrawal each time. This procedure should stop the baby getting the habit of suckling relentlessly and greedily. Otherwise there is a risk that she will gulp down quantities of milk and air much more quickly than is good for her.

Colic

A number of homoeopathic remedies are useful in treating colic. For bad-tempered babies, whose colic is worse between 4 and 8 pm, give Lycopodium. To those who appear to be doubled up with pain and seem better lying on their stomachs, give a dose of Colocynthis (*see Part Three, page 145*).

Mild Infections

Sometimes a slight conjunctivitis – an inflammation of the eyes – may result from contact with mucus in the birth canal during delivery.

Aromatherapy for Colic and Crying

Where to Use	Essential Oils	How to Use
Baby's room	Neroli, Roman chamomile	1–2 drops in a diffuser or on a cotton wool ball
On baby	Roman chamomile, mandarin	To 30ml almond oil, add 2 drops Roman chamomile or 1 drop Roman chamomile and 1 drop mandarin. Massage abdomen, clockwise
On baby's feet	Roman chamomile, mandarin	To 30ml almond oil, add 2 drops Roman chamomile or 1 drop Roman chamomile and 1 drop mandarin. Massage baby's feet (*see page 77*)

This may be treated with homoeopathic remedies, available from a qualified practitioner. While the baby has catarrhal discharges, whether from the nose or ears, the mother should avoid dairy food and refined carbohydrates, especially sugar.

Nappy Rash

This may occur if the stools and urine change composition through incomplete digestion. If breast-feeding, you should review your own diet. It may be that you need to exchange anything very salty, sugary, spicy or pickled for blander food.

Watch for other signs of distress that may result from an unsettled or broken routine, such as irregular feeds, too much travel, or a change of environment.

Use a little Calendula cream on the areas that seem to be most sensitive. The homoeopathic remedy, Sulphur, can often be useful for curing nappy rash.

The Herbal Options

Purpose	Herb	How to Use
To prevent sore nipples	Rosewater, honey, marigold or chamomile cream, almond oil	Apply to nipples after feeding
To reduce congestion or engorgement of breasts	Cleavers, marigold, dandelion root	Mother takes internally
To enhance mother's immune system in order to ward off infection in baby	Chamomile, ginger, cinnamon, thyme, echinacea, lemon balm	Mother takes internally
To relax baby's gut and help prevent colic	Chamomile, dill, fennel, lemon balm, cardamom, hops	Mother takes internally or bathes baby with infusion or decoction added to bath water
To avoid or ease nappy rash	Lavender, chamomile, marigold or thyme, rosewater	Wash baby's bottom with infusion, or apply as cream
To treat thrush	Calendula cream, powdered golden seal	Mother washes affected area with dilute cider vinegar or thyme infusion and applies herbs
To reduce parental fatigue	Equal amounts of Chinese angelica, ginger, nettles and false unicorn root	Mother takes internally
To help relieve sleepless nights (as a tonic)	Skullcap, vervain, wild oats, ginseng, licorice, rosemary	Mother takes internally
To reduce frustration	Bach flower remedies: holly and impatiens	Mother takes internally
To reduce apprehension	Bach flower remedies: aspen and mimulus	Mother takes internally
To improve sleeping and eating patterns	Bach flower remedy: walnut	Mother takes internally

Your Baby's Structural Development

Your baby's physical growth needs a firm structural base on which to develop. If this is established at an early age then a good foundation is set.

At this stage, the osteopath is looking for asymmetries of structure, restrictions of movement, and tightness or lack of mobility in the spine, the neck, the pelvis, the hips or any of the joints; also for weakness in the muscular and soft-tissue structures.

Digestive disorders are among many that may be helped by osteopathy through the release of restriction. There is a vital two-way interaction between musculo-skeletal structure and the function of the internal organs. Structural restrictions, particularly in the thoracic spine, may impede the workings of the digestive organs, causing wind, colic, constipation, diarrhoea, blockage, pressure, or pain or discomfort.

Even where the digestive condition has no structural cause, it will still reflect into the structure, indicating the presence and location of visceral disturbance. It can be treated osteopathically via the structure, in order to influence the stomach, pylorus, intestines or other organs within.

Visceral osteopathic techniques can also be gently applied to the abdominal organs in order to relieve tensions and spasms which may be causing colic and discomfort.

Restrictions in the upper thoracic spine and thorax may lead to respiratory difficulties or predispose to asthma and can be eased by articulation and soft-tissue treatment.

Infectious conditions can also be helped by encouraging lymphatic drainage through the use of soft-tissue massage along lymphatic pathways, and also through applying lymphatic pump techniques.

The Cranio-sacral Check

By two weeks, remoulding is usually complete, in so far as it is going to occur naturally, and the baby is usually settling into whatever patterns of behaviour will prevail.

At this stage – any time from two weeks onwards and not too long after – it is advisable for the baby to have a cranio-sacral check-up, even if the birth went smoothly. Many conditions, such as epilepsy, autism, dyslexia, learning difficulties and squint, may be due to minor distortions of the cranium at birth, but may only emerge many years later.

A simple check-up can guard against these conditions. If there is anything wrong, it can, at this stage, usually be resolved fairly quickly, whereas later it might never reach complete resolution. In any case, treatment at this stage can remove the minor distortions that probably affect all of us to some degree and ensure the happiest baby, with maximum potential.

Firstly, the therapist is likely to check the overall quality of the cranio-sacral system, the power and energy of its motion, the state of tension or ease of the body, and the overall characteristics of the cranio-sacral system and the baby generally. This should include checking the grip and the sucking reflex. The therapist will also look and feel for symmetry within the cranium and in the body as a whole, through light contact on various parts of the body, especially:

1 *The Pelvis* Being large relative to other parts of the body, this is easily distorted during its twisting passage through the birth canal. Pelvic distortion may lead to back pain, sciatica, hip, knee and lower limb problems, and osteoarthritis later in life. It is especially important in female babies, whose child-bearing ability may be affected by pelvic asymmetries.

2 *The Abdomen, Thorax and Diaphragm* Birth is a natural process but nature is by no means perfect, nor does every birth go smoothly. The process is nearly always arduous for both mother and baby. Indeed for the baby, being pushed through the narrow birth canal is almost inevitably traumatic to some degree.

The stresses of birth often accumulate particularly in the area of the solar plexus, with consequent tightness and tension in the diaphragm, the stomach, the pylorus and the surrounding digestive organs. It is very common to find tension and stress here in babies, especially those who have undergone a difficult birth. This is one of the main areas contributing to colic, regurgitation, poor feeding, abdominal pain, discomfort, pulling up knees into the abdomen, crying, and screaming.

3 *The Cranial Base* This takes most of the compressive strain of being pushed through the birth canal. It is the area through which many vital structures pass, connecting head to body and body to head. Compression in this area can lead to a variety of symptoms and conditions including hyperactivity and behavioural disorders; weakness, floppiness, low energy, poor sucking reflex, breathing difficulties, headache and migraine, digestive disturbances, colic, poor feeding and regurgitation.

4 *The Neck* The neck is often found to be retracted or pulled back following birth trauma, or it might turn more easily to one side than to the other. This may be due to compression of the neck and base of the skull. Arching of the back is also a common sign of discomfort brought on by specific problems.

5 *The Cranium* Any distortion or compression of the cranium may have repercussions directly affecting the brain, or may interfere with blood supply to the brain, the nerves emerging from the brain, the membranes surrounding the brain, or the cerebro-spinal fluid which bathes, supplies and protects the brain. The brain is, of course, fundamental to all other functions in the body, and so proper integration of the cranium and brain function is vital for your baby's optimum health and happiness.

The cranio-sacral therapist is also likely to enquire about your baby's breathing patterns, sleep patterns, lying preferences, any asymmetries of movement or behaviour or any other concerns you may have. In identifying the cause of any problems affecting the baby, the therapist will also take into account the emotional state of the baby (which may in turn be closely related to that of the mother), and the baby's environment, family relations, nutritional factors, allergies, medication, and any accidents, injuries, infections or illnesses.

Considering the Mother

It is also important to consider the mother's welfare. At this stage she is likely to be exhausted by the combination of the birth process, constant baby care, and feeding at all times of the day and night with no opportunity for proper sleep and relaxation. She may find that she is too busy looking after the new baby even to take stock of her own condition.

It must be emphasized that the baby's welfare is also dependent on the well-being of the parents. Most mothers neglect themselves – and are also neglected by others. This can cause them to suffer further ill effects, whether post-natal depression, or physical and emotional difficulties later in life.

Cranio-sacral therapy can play an integral part in looking after the mothe, and ensuring that she will be encouraged at all costs to take time off for treatment, rest, and exercises, and generally caring for herself.

Your Baby's Playtime

Some time after a feed, but not directly, have fun with your baby in creative movement. See how she loves you to sing, talk, blow on her hands, and nibble her fingers. Enjoy that divine baby smell.

Below left and below. *Hold your baby over your shoulder, pat her gently, and rock. You will both enjoy the soothing sensation. Put her across your knees; if it feels safer, sit cross-legged on the bed. Rock her, tilting her gently up and down. Smile and talk to her.*

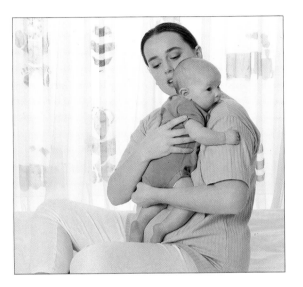

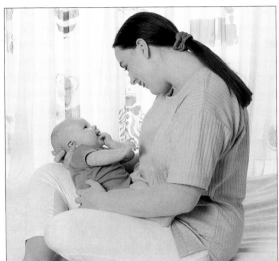

Right and inset. *Lay the baby on her back. Hold her hands (your thumb in her palms) and feel the strong grip. Massage her hands and arms and pretend to pull her upwards. Babies hang on and almost brace themselves for the lift. Support her head and tug her towards you. Cross her arms over her chest and then place them flat at her sides — now move them up and down slowly. Tell her what you are doing.*

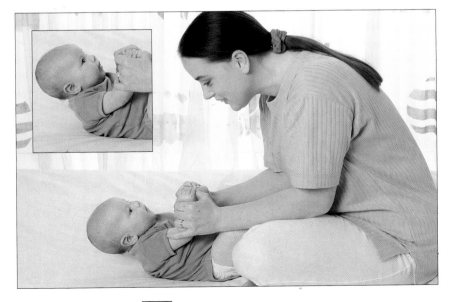

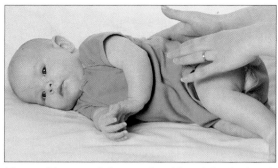

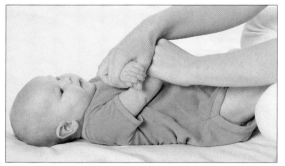

Above. *Turn your baby on to her side, rub her back and round her into the foetal position. Now turn her over. Babies soon recognize the sensation when you turn their knees. Watch the head follow round in perfect alignment.*

Above. *Hold her hands under her thumbs. Bring the hands across her chest – then gently squeeze and release them. Cup her head in your hands and warm it – stroke her cheeks meanwhile with your thumb.*

Right. *Put her on her back and hold her legs with thumbs behind her knees. Lift her bottom just off the bed* (top inset). *Bounce her once or twice, then push her knees up against her chest* (bottom inset) *and roll her gently from side to side* (main picture). *Rub her feet with your thumbs on the soles and work up to her knees. Her head will be alarmingly floppy, so when you pick her up, always support it.*

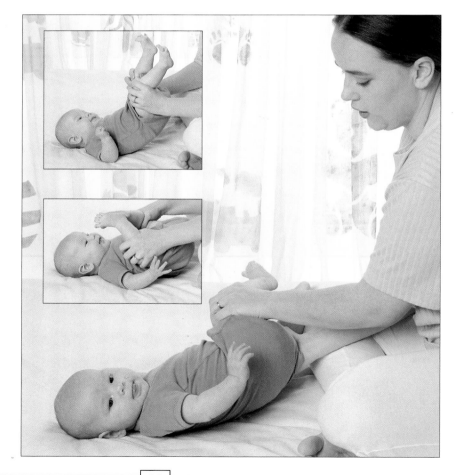

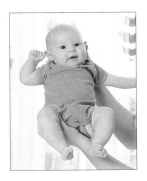

Left. *Support your baby's head as you lift her like a tray – up, down. Then swing her to and fro on her tummy.*

Right. *Take the baby's weight so that she presses with her toes. She will try to knee-bob or even walk.*

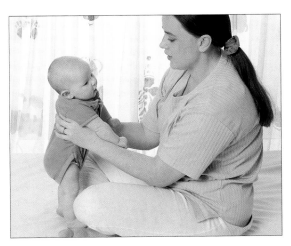

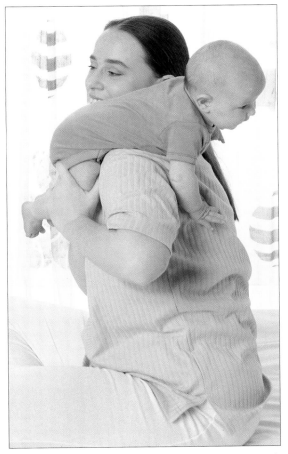

Above. *Play at rocking in a strong swinging motion and, holding the baby's legs firmly, tip her over your shoulder in a fireman's lift. Hold her by the hips and tip her upside down against your back.*

By the time your baby is six weeks old, she will recognize her movement playtime, and as she grows stronger she will increase the energy level, so your lifts and drops can be a little more rapid and unexpected.

By eight weeks she will love being pulled up by her hands into a sitting position. Hold her head fairly firmly and rock her. Lift and tilt her up from lying on her back by her feet. 'Walk' her legs up and down – she will smile with pleasure and gurgle at you.

Hold her hips and tip her upside down, stretching her back. Roll her back, gently giving her time to follow.

Babies love bopping, so put on some music and dance together holding her in your arms. You will be rewarded by a more profound sense of bonding and the recognition of love that every parent longs for – a delicious smile.

Towards three months old, your child will have changed almost beyond recognition. She is now able to 'socialize', smiling and burbling at you directly, and often at some length.

One result of this is that any attention you show her is likely to be rewarded in kind, with a delighted display of further affection from your newly expressive baby.

CHAPTER THREE

A Bundle of Joy

T he delightful stage of babyhood from three to six months is often over all too quickly; take every opportunity to relish it while you can.

Your baby will be reaching an age when minor ailments become commonplace. These are always a source of anxiety but in most cases there is no cause for concern. Of course you will want to relieve your baby's distress, and several ways to do this are described in the Conditions and Illnesses section in Part Three. You can be assured that many acute symptoms indicate the body's defences at work as the infant develops immunity.

The objectives of naturopathic treatment are to relieve discomfort and create conditions for the self-healing processes to work. One feature of this approach is that you seldom need resort to antibiotics or medicines such as aspirin or Calpol which suppress the healing response.

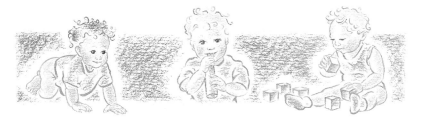

Common Problems

Colic and Digestive Discomfort

With severe colic it may be helpful to substitute a breast feed with a bottle of dill water: simmer a dessertspoon of dill seed in hot water, then strain and give by bottle at a comfortable temperature. Dill water may also be given between feeds to relieve colic. Alternatively, seek the help of a homoeopath or cranio-sacral therapist (*see also Part Three, pages 144–5*).

Catarrhal Infections and Rashes

Bottle feeds should contain no sugar or other sweet foods. Do not give citrus juices if your baby has nappy rash or any other skin rash.

Avoid cow's milk products and use soya infant formula instead.

Homoeopathic remedies may prove beneficial, too, for these conditions (*see also Part Three, pages 141 and 154*).

Teething

Your baby will probably start to teethe at around five to six months. Homoeopathic remedies to relieve this state include Chamomilla, Calcarea carbonica and Pulsatilla. Light massage may also provide some relief, particularly so with an aromatic oil (*see Aromatherapy Solutions below*).

Aromatherapy Solutions

Problem	Essential Oils	How to Use
Colic	Chamomile	Add 1 drop to 20ml milk and mix into baby's bathwater
Crying	Chamomile	Add 1 drop to 20ml milk and mix into baby's bathwater
Parental fatigue	Lemon	Add 4–5 drops of oil to eggcup of boiling water. Have it beside you as you work or relax. The aromatic vapour will keep you from falling asleep and clear your thoughts
Teething	Lavender and Roman chamomile	To 30ml sweet almond oil (the carrier), add 1 drop each of the essential oils and massage along baby's jawline
	Lavender	Add 1 drop to baby's bathwater

The Power of Touch

The benefits of massage for babies between three and six months old are both profound and numerous. Your baby's development, both physical and mental, is proceeding apace. She will now be lying on her belly, lifting her head up and holding her upper body weight on her arms while turning her head to take in more of her surroundings. The head will be much more steady when she is helped to sit up.

Your baby is using her hands more, watching them and showing a desire to grasp things. She has probably discovered she can roll over from her tummy on to her back. Laying your baby on her side will help her cope with rolling as she gets used to the change of perspective.

Some babies at six months are sitting, supported, for some time.

She will be showing obvious signs of pleasure: making sounds, thrashing her arms and legs about and, at around four months old, laughing out loud – a delightful sound.

Most babies are feeding on solids and showing preferences for certain foods. All are developing their personalities and making their needs and wants known to their parents.

Massage is a fun part of your baby's routine and can be extended to include some exercises for limbs and back. Now that your baby is older, her massage can also be expanded to repeat each stage at least three or four times (*see pages 76–8*).

To work her left arm, use your right hand and vice versa. Stroke the arm from wrist to shoulder, over the shoulder and down. Work up the forearm from wrist to elbow, then work the upper arm from elbow to shoulder, always with a slight squeeze.

On the feet, massage each toe with a slight squeeze and rolling movement.

Massage is a powerful medium for enhancing your baby's development and deepening the bond between baby and parent. The use of aromatic oils adds to the experience.

Below. Open out your baby's hand and circle into the palm with your thumb. Massage each finger, pressing and rolling it between your thumb and fingers.

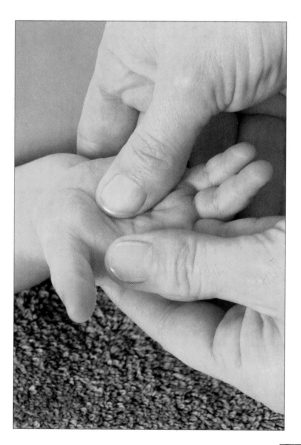

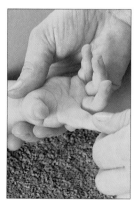

Left. In massaging your baby's hands, give a slight stretch to each finger.

Below. Massage the foot using your thumbs. Circle over the top of the baby's foot, then into the sole of the foot. Massage each toe with a slight squeeze and rolling movement and with a little stretch for each toe.

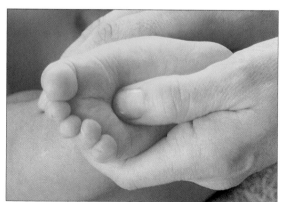

Face Massage

Not all babies enjoy face massage. Also they do not keep their heads still for very long and care is needed to avoid the eyes.

Right. *Gently place your hands around the baby's head.*

Below. *Massage scalp, taking extra care of softer parts.*

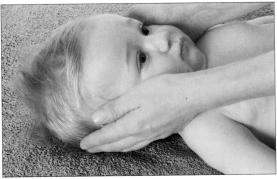

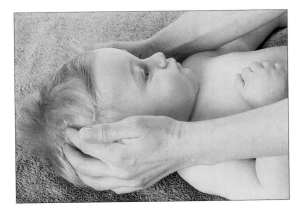

Below, upper left. *Use your thumbs to massage across the cheeks from the nose out to the ears.*

Below, bottom left. *Use your fingertips to circle over the baby's cheeks. This will probably cause lots of dribble. In young babies it may also cause them to look for a feed.*

Below. *Glide your thumbs along the chin, keeping them just under the jawbone.*

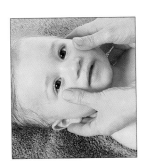

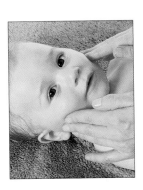

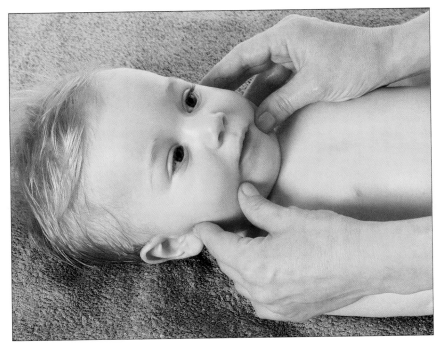

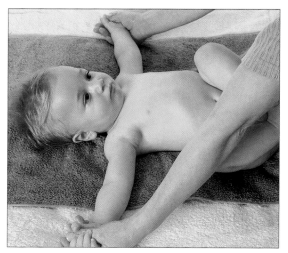

Above. *Lie the baby on his back. Take each of his hands and open out his arms until they are fully extended.*

Right. *Bring the arms to cross over the chest. Extend them and repeat. Alternate which arm is on top.*

Strengthening Your Baby's Back Muscles after Massage

The exercises on this page will help your baby's subsequent coordination. Never push against resistance, but follow any lead and describe what you do, counting or using directions like 'open', 'stretch', 'close', and making it fun. Repeat each movement three times.

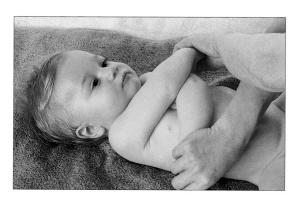

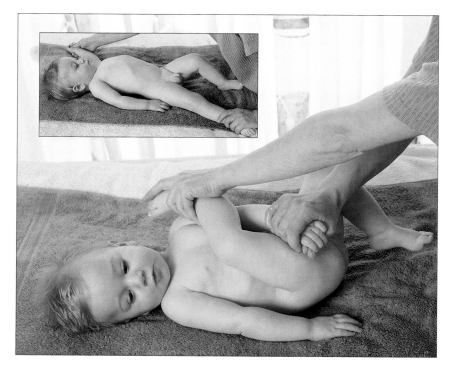

Left inset. *Take your baby's left arm and right leg and extend them away from the body. Make encouraging sounds as you gently stretch the limbs, monitoring his responses all the time.*

Left. *Bring the left arm and right leg towards each other until the right leg is by the left shoulder and the left arm/hand is by the right buttock. Extend again. Repeat for the right arm and left leg. Never risk forcing the joints of the hip or shoulder, and be aware of the position of the knee and ankle.*

Your Baby's Perception

Between three and four months of age, babies are able, on their own, to disengage their attention from objects. It is at this age that they choose what they want to look at and explore. As well as using colour in clothing, it is important, at this stage in the child's development, to surround her with colour.

One way of doing this is in the choice of colours used to decorate the room where she sleeps. Designated tints should be used for this room; that is, colours with 50 per cent white added to them. All of these colours tend to blend harmoniously, even if they are opposites on the spectrum wheel (*see below*). Choose a pastel-coloured wallpaper which displays an interesting design of toys or animals; for example there is often wonderful wallpaper on the market which is covered in teddy bears performing all manner of antics. The curtains can be selected to match the background colour of the wallpaper. Lampshades can be purchased with dolls and toys, dressed in a variety of colours, suspended beneath them. When toys are distributed elsewhere in the room, they create endless visual enjoyment.

Up until the age of six months, babies lack the coordination needed to reach out and grasp an object. Also, their hand muscles have not developed sufficiently to be able to do this. They will make swiping movements at objects within their reach, sometimes managing to touch them but more frequently not. A multi-coloured mobile hung over the cot will not only provide visual stimulation but will also help develop the infant's ability to reach and grasp. Another possibility would be a variety of coloured objects or toys strung across the cot.

Following the Bates method, you can continue to amplify and extend the movement of your baby's eyes. Introduce palming for short periods by holding your hands lightly over your baby's eyes, while singing and chatting to her. You can also extend the range of procedures (*see pages 43–6 with the additional exercises shown below*).

It is reassuring to remember that sight during infancy is very variable, and if, during a clinical check, your baby's sight appears deficient, it is worth waiting a week to re-check if the same defect is still present, or whether it has already changed.

With your baby, play with toys and roll a soft ball towards her. Let her reach out for things and allow her to wriggle on the floor. Recovery from parental fatigue can be assisted by setting aside short periods for yourself for relaxation and palming. Think through and review difficulties using ESR (*see, in Part One, the kinesiology section, exercise 2, on page 43*).

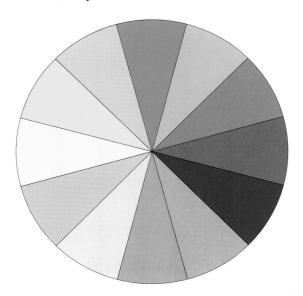

Left. *The twelve standard colours with 50 per cent white added. These pastels, or 'designated' tints, blend harmoniously even when they are opposites on the wheel.*

Become open to all-round sensory awareness: let your sight become active and let your hearing take in the sounds of your environment. When you go for a walk, tune in to the rustling of the leaves and the chatter of the birds.

• After four months, let the baby have plastic blocks and other clean harmless objects that she can put in her mouth, since this is an essential way of gaining experience and learning about the things in the world.

• Give your baby opportunities to move around, by providing a safe area on the floor. There she can move and eventually crawl in order to experience size, space and distance. The more her chance of unhampered physical exercise, the surer her movements will become.

• Avoid baby walkers and try not to rely unduly on the use of baby chairs, both of which can hinder integrated left–right and binocular visual development.

• Use the emotional stress release (*see kinesiology exercise 2, on page 43*) to diminish any visual as well as emotional tension.

• Ensure that there are plenty of coloured objects around to stimulate your baby's interest in the visible world.

• Every day, take your baby into the open air, ideally bright sunshine, so that she can be nourished by full-spectrum light.

• Smile and laugh, speak and sing, to allow sound to become integrated with sight.

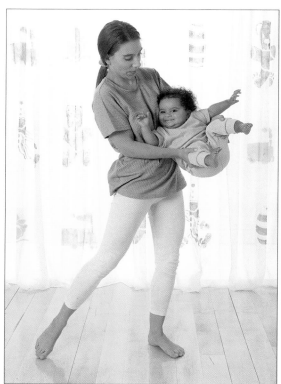

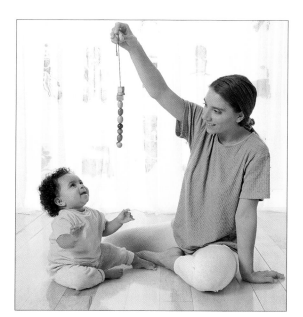

Above. *As your baby becomes old enough to sit unsupported and move her head more freely, she finds it easier to look around her. Wave something bright and colourful, like a flower or a string of wooden beads, to help stimulate her interest in visual movement.*

Above. *Hold your baby with her back to your body, and rhythmically swing around or sway from side to side. Bounce her gently up and down. As she gets older, you can increase the vigour and range of movement. This helps to develop the coordinated natural movements of the eyes.*

Parental Fatigue

Babyhood can be one of the most stressful times for both parents. Simple Alexander technique procedures, such as lying on the floor and increasing your awareness, and consciously releasing muscular tension, can be very successful in alleviating tiredness (*see Part One, pages 51–3*). A course of lessons at this time can be invaluable because by moving in more efficient ways, many parents would feel they had more energy.

Other Benefits of the Alexander Technique

• Learning easier ways to lift and carry your child. This will also be more comfortable for the baby.
• Learning to push prams and carry portable car seats without unnecessary strain.
• Not reacting with tension when your baby cries. Tension causes fatigue.
• Holding your baby with active consciousness and realizing how precious she is: a source of new-found energy for both parents.
• Helping to take each day as it comes rather than being anxious about whether you are being a good mother or father.

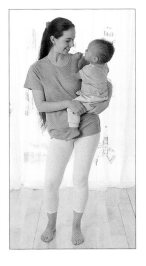 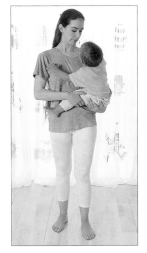

Above. *Many mothers support their baby on the hip while standing. This may lead to lower back pain and put the body out of alignment.*

Above, right. *For improved posture, give both feet equal weight in supporting your baby.*

Right and far right. *Pushing a buggy is stressful if you have poor posture. Be as upright as possible, with head balanced above the spine.*

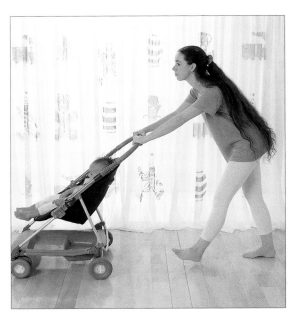 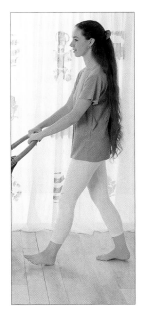

Your Baby's Structural Development

As your baby develops, patterns of movement and symmetry become clearer and any imbalances should be addressed immediately. The sooner they are treated, the more completely they can be resolved.

As your baby starts to sit unsupported, the osteopath will be looking for the development of normal curvature of the spine and to guard against any lateral curvature (scoliosis), a tendency to lean to one side, or any difficulties in sitting upright.

Establishing good postural patterns starts at the earliest opportunity. If posture is allowed to go wrong now, it may never improve. Spinal curvature and postural patterns may lead not only to back problems, but also to effects on the internal organs, causing digestive, pelvic or respiratory disturbances and may also influence your child's subsequent mobility, agility and coordination.

Gently swinging your baby by the feet can be very useful, as well as being highly enjoyable for most babies. It provides an excellent opportunity to examine the spine in a fully extended and straightened position (which is often difficult with squirming, wriggling babies). It gives the body a good stretch, opening up the joints and soft tissues, and revealing the areas that are reluctant to open up and stretch. It also carries a healthy rush of arterial blood to the head. Swinging is something that can be carried out by parents at home, though always carefully, sensitively, gently and not for too long at one time.

The Cranio-sacral Check

A cranio-sacral check-up once a month is advisable at this delicate age. If the baby has not yet been checked by a cranio-sacral therapist, every effort should be made to have this

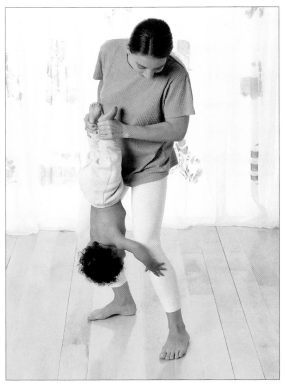

Above. *Hold your baby securely around her ankles and swing gently from side to side. Most small children love this. Only do it if they are enjoying themselves, and then for a maximum of half a minute at a time.*

done by the age of six months, before the bones ossify and structural patterns become imprinted and ingrained.

Problems Addressed

• *Ear Infections* are common at this age, along with glue ear, deafness, and infections of the nose and throat. So too are digestive disturbances and colds. All are helped by cranio-sacral therapy since it can be used to strengthen the immune system, and to improve arterial and venous blood flow and lymphatic flow, thereby enabling the body to deal with the infection. This is particularly applicable to ear infections, which are often due to blockage of the auditory tube (or Eustachian tube) which drains the middle ear.

• *Asymmetries of Eye Movement* are common in the early months but by now they should have settled; any indication of a persistent squint should be investigated. Squints can be due to a variety of causes affecting the bones which form the orbit, the muscles of the eye, or the cranial nerves supplying these muscles. Cranio-sacral therapy can be very effective at treating squints at an early age. It is important to treat not only the specific structures of the eye, but also to identify pulls, twists, and tensions anywhere in the system that may be contributing to the condition.

• *Digestive Problems* Colicky symptoms often fade at around three months, but underlying causes should still be identified. Reactions to changes in diet need to be taken into account. A healthy, comfortable digestive system will normally cope with these changes. Reactions are often due to tensions and stresses held in the digestive organs and solar plexus, but cranio-sacral therapy can help release these.

• *Teething Problems* may be helped, and discomfort minimized, with cranio-sacral treatment.

• *Asymmetries of the Neck (torticollis)*, with the head held to one side, are often an indication of underlying restrictions. This condition is often operated on if severe, but it is very effectively treated by the gentler, non-invasive methods of cranio-sacral therapy.

Your Baby's Playtime

Some babies are mini-athletes by now. They have swiftly become very aware of new movement sensations. They also love sharing them. All the old rhyming games are fun for them – and for you: the baby can focus on your face, smile and chuckle.

Far right and right. *Sit your baby on your lap and play all the familiar nursery games. These can include such things as pretending to ride a horse or fly through the air, or doing drops through your knees. Any games and songs that interest and stimulate will not only delight her but build her confidence.*

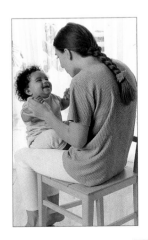

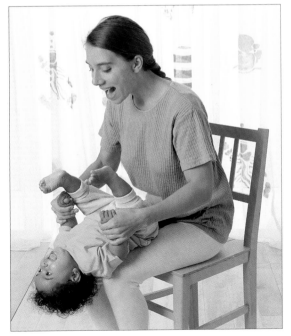

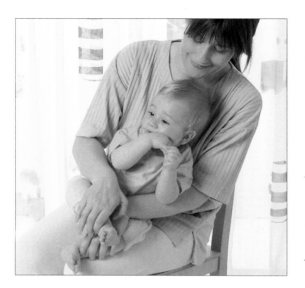

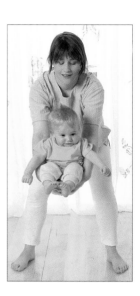

Left. *In playing traditional rhyming games, babies love the rhythm long before they understand the words.*

Right. *Rock him gently to and fro and then swing him more vigorously. As you do so, pretend to throw him up. 'Throw' him up and across to a partner – a lovely game. Be very sensitive to his feelings about how energetic you should be.*

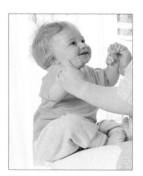

Above and right. *Holding your baby by his hands or under his arms, help him into an upright position and allow him to 'stand' and pad his feet. Bounce him up and down: he'll laugh and gurgle with pleasure. When supported in this way he will constantly try to sit or stand. If necessary, prop him up on cushions in order to help him see around more freely.*

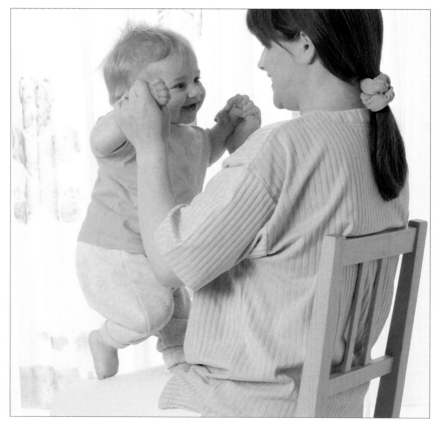

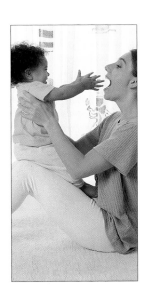

Left and below. *Sit with your knees bent and place your baby on top, supporting her under the arms. Drop your knees to the floor, holding on to her to ease the jolt (below, inset). Then rock her back and forth on your outstretched legs (below, main picture).*

Right. *Put her on top of your head (like a cushion) and turn her slowly from side to side.*

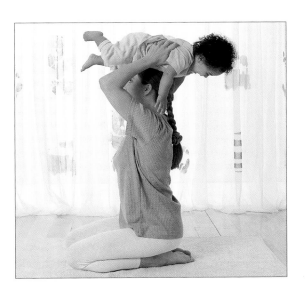

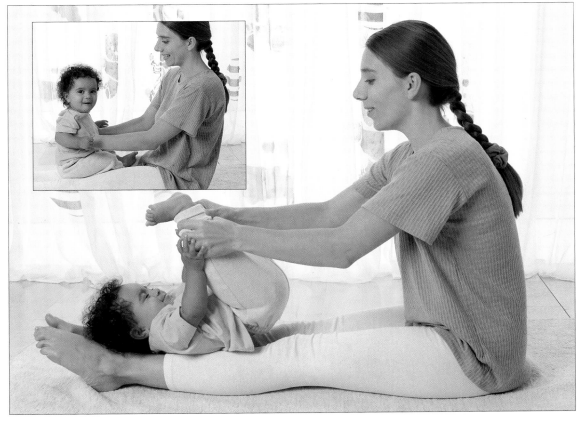

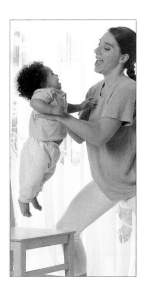
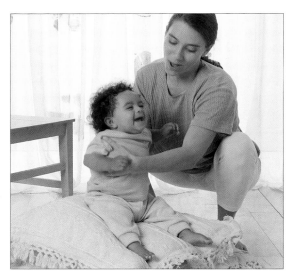

Left. *Play the 'jumps'. Swing your baby up, holding her under the arms, and perch her on a chair* (far left). *Then swing her off to a table, the floor or window sill, making noises as she flies through the air. Lift her on to your shoulders, then support her back and walk about. Swing her down through your knees – and up. Children love this, right up to when they are too heavy to lift.*

As part of your baby's playtime, put down a towel or baby mat and give her time to kick without a nappy. She might like a few minutes on her tummy, though some babies hate this even when they can hold up their heads.

Throughout her second three months hands are becoming important. Help her hold a ball, and let her feel a cushion and touch your cheek or hair. Play 'pat-a-cake' and 'clap hands' (up and down is easier than sideways). Dangle a toy for her to stretch out to and pat and catch.

She can also follow your voice. Try giving little surprises: 'Cuckoo' – 'Peek-a-boo'.

Bath time should be fun. Allow lots of time, and let the baby kick against your hand. Splash her hands about. Before dressing her, let her play on the bath mat. If you roll her over onto her tummy she may try to push forward, so help by stretching our her legs.

Hand–eye coordination continues to develop fast; she will be fascinated by new colours and textiles and any new shapes. Play hideaway games – tucking a cup, ball, dolly under or behind your back or blanket – where is it? She will stretch out for it and even hold it briefly. This game will help develop her visual coordination as well as being simply fun.

Keep all her games going; she'll have quite a repertoire of tricks by now. For example, to play 'swinging basket', lie your baby down on her back, hold her hands and feet together and pull her up slowly, then give a little swing.

By now, at the end of her first six months, your child's capacity for enjoyment in play will be expanding at an ever greater rate. She has become self-confident and has gained a real sense of fun.

Her range of communication can sometimes seem to be greater every day. She may show anger when a toy is taken away, but she can be easily distracted by a new object. Generally she shows eagerness and anger vocally and by facial expression and arm and body movements. Sometimes she shows anxiety towards strangers by frowning and withdrawal; mostly, however, her friendliness and curiosity combine to make her a delight.

Playtime is when you and your partner can really enjoy her company and deepen the bond that already exists.

CHAPTER FOUR

Growing Up and Out

❧

Your baby will develop rapidly in the second six months. By now she will be quite vocal, uttering squeals and screams of pleasure and disapproval. She will be able to sit for short periods without being supported. Everything that goes on will fascinate her and her vision will be developing rapidly. Your baby's environment, both visual and acoustic, is vital to healthy physical development.

Emotional development is just as important as physique. In addition to wanting companionship, she will start to demand independence. Give her freedom to kick and roll about safely, and later to crawl and try to walk. At nine months, as her memory develops, she may recognize familiar preparations for bathtime or meals, and briefly wait for attention. Appreciating these changes, and adjusting to your baby's emotional development, is vital to a good parental relationship.

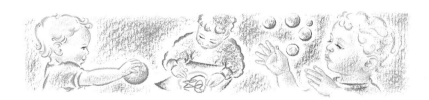

Common Problems

Teething

Strengthen the gums by giving your baby hard objects to bite on, including a raw carrot or a piece of apple. If you cannot get organic carrots, scrape or scrub well to get rid of pesticides. The stress of teething may often precipitate catarrhal disorders. If teething problems persist, follow the advice given in Chapter Three (*see page 155*).

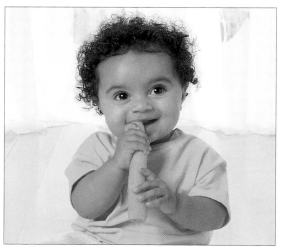

Above. *Give your baby a raw carrot or piece of apple to bite on to toughen the gums. When teeth appear, watch for fragments of food which might lodge in the throat.*

Catarrhal Conditions

Snuffles and catarrhal discharges may call for some modification of diet if you are introducing more bottle feeds and solids. Use puréed fruits and vegetables only, or juices, for several days (*see Naturopathy in Part One, page 10*). If you are still breast-feeding, review your own diet to exclude dairy products and refined carbohydrates for a few days.

Herbs to Treat Infection

Herbs can be given directly to the baby to help ward off or treat infections that siblings may be bringing into the house. These include:
• Garlic, an effective antiseptic which can be cooked with food. Other antiseptic and immune-enhancing herbs can be mixed with food, such as thyme, rosemary, oregano, fennel, and sage, and given as teas. These include chamomile, thyme, hyssop, lemon balm, and St John's wort.
• Echinacea, of which you can give 5 drops in a teaspoon or two of boiled water to prevent and treat infections.
• Nettles and dandelion leaves; these can be added to soups in small amounts, to enhance nutrition and act as general tonics.

Weaning

Solids can now be introduced. Some children find it hard to be weaned and the Bach flower remedy, walnut, can be helpful at this stage.

The child's innate dislikes and likes of certain foods are becoming evident and allergies may show themselves as new foods are added to her accustomed diet. These ailments can be treated homoeopathically.

The Power of Touch

Continue loving contact with your baby through regular massage, as described in the sequences in previous chapters. You will be familiar with your baby's little body contours, her muscle tone will be more developed, and she will appear quite plump and cuddlesome.

You can now add new exercises for her legs and hips to encourage sitting and standing.

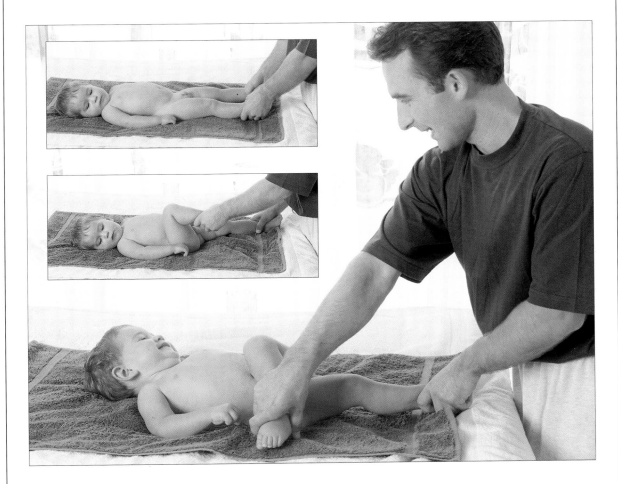

Top, inset. *With the baby lying on his back, hold each leg just over the ankles.*

Middle, inset. *Bend one leg at the knee towards the chest while almost straightening the other. Change legs and repeat the movement three or four times. Open the knees and bring the soles of the baby's feet together. With knees open, lift the feet towards the tummy. As long as your baby is comfortable, you can extend this stretch by taking the feet further up the body.*

Above. *With knee bent, take the baby's foot across the tummy to the opposite hip, then straighten again. Repeat with the other leg. Do both legs three or four times.*

Points to Remember

- *Massage will make your baby hungry and thirsty, so ideally the sequence will be: massage, bath, feed, bed.*
- *If you have been massaging regularly you will know which parts your baby likes best and how much pressure she finds comfortable.*
- *It's never too late to start massage.*
- *Baby massage can benefit all the major systems of your baby's body.*
- *Loving touch relaxes your baby, leading to a deep and restful sleep.*

Aromatherapy Solutions

Problem	Essential Oils	How to Use
Parental fatigue	Mandarin	5 drops essential oil to 10ml any carrier oil (such as almond or jojoba) for foot massage
Teething	Chamomile	Use in warm compress held against baby's jawline. Renew as it cools
	Chamomile or lavender	Add 1–2 drops to vaporizer for use in baby's room
Tantrums	Chamomile, neroli, lavender or mandarin	Vaporize oil in baby's room before the nap
	Neroli or mandarin	Add 1 drop to baby's bathwater. Dilute in milk as described on page 23
	Neroli or mandarin	Add 1 drop to 30ml almond carrier oil and give baby a body massage
For parent after baby's tantrum	Neroli or ylang ylang	Add 2 drops to 10ml almond oil, rub a little on to wrists and inhale

Parental Fatigue

Erratic and inadequate meals can be a major cause of chronic fatigue. The breast-feeding mother needs regular fuel from high-quality nutrients. Blood-sugar levels can fluctuate dramatically at times of extra physical and emotional demand, such as childbirth and breast-feeding.

Make sure you have well-balanced main meals that provide enough protein or complex carbohydrate to sustain you. If you experience fatigue, it may help to have a light savoury snack between meals and last thing at night. A handful or two of nuts or seeds, for example sunflower or pumpkin, or a rice biscuit with cottage cheese or a savoury spread such as yeast extract, miso, or pâté, can usually provide top-up energy to keep you going.

The savoury meals release their energy slowly and last longer. Avoid sweet and sugary snacks and drinks as these make the tiredness worse in the long run, by interfering with the body's energy-producing mechanism.

Your Baby's Perception

This is the period in an infant's life when she learns to sit unsupported, leaving her hands free to explore and reach out for desired objects. It is also the age when babies begin to observe and explore their surroundings and seek things out.

Interest in the colours preferred by babies goes back to the turn of the century. Because babies are unable to answer questions, their preferences are inferred from their behaviour. In one experiment, four-month-old infants were shown different colours one at a time,

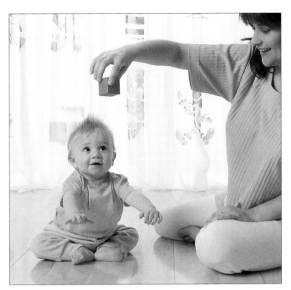

Above. *Interest is essential to encouraging a baby's tracking, focusing and coordinative abilities. Here, an attractively coloured brick is a source of attention.*

Developing Sight

You can help the development of your baby's vision, through the Bates method:

• Encourage crawling and avoid constricting aids such as baby walkers.

• Help your baby to negotiate stairs.

• Introduce coordinated play, like pat-a-cake.

• Make sounds together.

• Supply suitable things for your baby to touch. If possible, give objects she can safely explore by putting in her mouth.

• Avoid being over-rigid during baby tantrums and maintain firm boundaries.

• Play sight-following games and help to begin catching a soft ball.

• Help your child to focus, by playing finger-following games.

• Do your best to be extra supportive during weaning, since, for some children, this is a difficult transition.

In addition to these new elements of Bates for this age group, turn back and follow the exercises in Chapter Two (*see pages 83–4*) and Chapter Three (*see pages 97–8*), and below (*see pages 118–19*).

and each for about fifteen seconds. It was found that they chose to spend most time looking at red and blue. When a primary colour was shown alongside one that was blended, most babies looked longest at the pure colours. Another experiment was carried out by a psychologist on his nine-month-old daughter in which he gave her toys that were either green or red. He noted that each time he did this, she showed a strong preference for a red toy over a green one.

This is the age when infants start to prefer toys in bright colours rather than pastel shades. A box of building bricks in bright red, blue and yellow will be a source of delight and visual stimulation.

At first the infant will handle the bricks in a disorganized way and merely play at hitting them together. It is not until a later age that children will start working constructively with such toys.

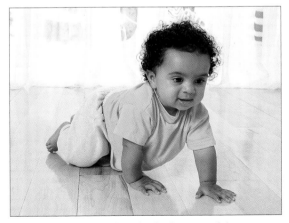

Above. *Crawling assists the development of the nervous system and body, from separated right and left use to both-sides-together functioning.*

Your Baby's Structural Development

As your baby starts to stand, crawl and walk, the structural patterns of development are further emphasized, and any aberrations or asymmetries in the way your baby moves should be dealt with by an osteopath.

It is not uncommon for one or both feet to be turned in. If this is mild, it may not appear to affect your baby immediately. But it may subsequently influence her mobility or coordination in running or jumping and may perhaps lead to falling over while learning to walk and starting to run.

Whilst this may be caused by a local problem in the foot, it is sometimes due to a more widespread structural pattern, reflecting up through the leg to the pelvis and the back, and will need to be balanced out by an osteopath.

Pelvic alignment is fundamental to structural balance as a whole and an important factor in subsequent back pain and hip and knee disorders. During sitting, such imbalances may not be evident, but they become so once your baby is standing.

So-called differences in leg length are often diagnosed, but mostly the cause is a pelvic imbalance. This needs to be put right at the level of the pelvis, the low back and the surrounding muscles and soft tissues.

It is helpful to observe your baby regularly during baths and while changing and playing. In this way you should be able to identify any structural asymmetries which can be resolved at this stage by an osteopath.

Understanding Your Child

The Alexander technique, while helping to combat parental tiredness, can also help you understand the way in which the human body is designed to move. It is fascinating to watch all the natural reflexes come into play as your child learns to crawl, balance when standing and take those first steps. Later you will notice that she loves all the physical sensations of running, jumping, kicking and throwing balls. During this stage, your child will pick up much of your own posture, and if you are conscious and careful of the way you move, she will be less likely to form harmful habits.

Once the parent appreciates the principles of good poise, he or she can avoid provoking poor coordination and bad posture. For example, many prams, pushchairs and car seats on the market today are badly designed and positively encourage slumping even at this early age. These are easy to spot once you know what to look for. It is common to see children struggling against backward-sloping seats in their determined efforts to maintain an upright posture. Sadly, parents can misinterpret this as being difficult, and chastise their children for perfectly innocent behaviour.

The Alexander technique can help you understand why your child behaves as she

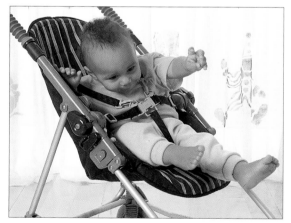

Above. *The backward-sloping shape of pushchairs and buggies are the first source of poor posture in adults. Here a child struggles to maintain his natural upright posture.*

does. This, in turn, will help you to be more patient when she makes the mistakes she needs to in order to learn certain lessons. You will be able to fulfil your role as your child's guardian without being over-protective.

The way in which we are treated in childhood, especially at this age, moulds us for the rest of our lives. A. S. Neil, one of the great educationalists of the twentieth century, once said there was no such thing as a problem child – only a problem parent. Many traumas that children experience could be overcome, given greater parental understanding.

As well as educating the body, the Alexander technique brings wider forms of understanding that make it invaluable in many forms of human relationship. The calmness you achieve when practising the technique not only helps you personally, but can thereby reduce stress levels throughout the family.

The Cranio-sacral Check

As your baby starts to crawl and stand up, it is helpful to observe the coordination of limbs and symmetry of movement, in case of any tendency to lean to one side or show incipient curvature of the spine. Any such problems can usually be treated effectively if caught early.

A cranio-sacral check-up every two to three months is advisable whenever the child has an illness, fall, or injury, or at any other time that you may be concerned about your baby.

Following any illness, such as a cold or an ear infection, babies (like adults) often seem not quite themselves for some time afterwards, remaining irritable, disgruntled and restless. This is often helped by cranio-sacral treatment clearing any lingering effects. Cranio-sacral therapy can also boost development of the immune system, ensuring optimum development and function of the thymus gland, the spleen, and the liver. Like others the immune system develops and gains strength through being exercised. Colds and minor infections are the challenges the body needs in order to develop strong immunity. They should not be regarded as entirely negative, to be suppressed and eradicated at all cost with medication, but rather as good exercise. Unnecessary antibiotics and other medication may undermine and weaken the development of the immune system. They are largely irrelevant to the majority of colds, which are mostly viral infections, whereas antibiotics are only effective against bacterial infections.

Any abnormalities of growth should by now be apparent. In particular, an exceptionally small head (which may be due to restriction of cranial bone mobility), or an exceptionally large one, can be treated effectively by cranio-sacral therapy. Headbanging and unusually forceful sucking may be the baby's attempt to release restrictions and discomfort within the cranium.

Treatment at this age takes on a new dimension, with your baby needing to be more entertained. Parents can contribute during treatment by ensuring that she is happily diverted and occupied.

Your Baby's Playtime

Your baby will be growing bigger and heavier by the day. You need to be very aware now of looking after your back – lifting a heavy child is a major hazard. Always bend your knees to pick her up, and pull in your tummy. Change hips when carrying her – avoid the habit of holding her always on one side rather than the other. Carry your baby on your back instead of in front if you are walking or standing for long.

Right. *To help your baby stretch, place his toys at the edge of his reach, and put him on his tummy. He will try to push with his knees. Gently pull him back to increase the stretch.*

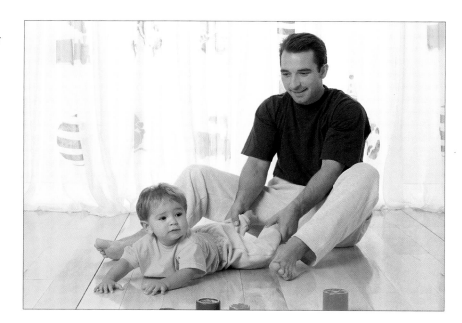

Below. *Lie on your back with your knees in the air. Holding your baby under the armpits, and perch him on your knees. Then, with plenty of warning, drop them or tilt him forward and bounce him on your tummy.*

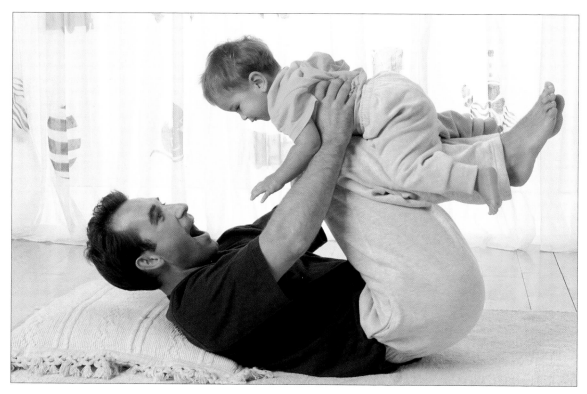

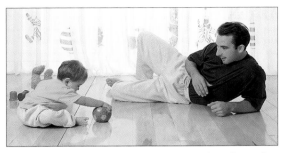

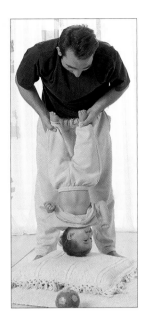

Above. *Let him play happily on his own but always be ready to join in. Babies can feel abandoned if left too long to play alone. Besides, when you join your baby, he will be getting the message that life is fun.*

Below. *Your baby will love being tickled, and playing hand and foot games – older children can play in this way with him, too. They are learning to relate and adjust to one another by laughing together.*

Left. *Hold his knees and gently turn him upside down. This stretches his back. He will turn his head and be intrigued by the new view. Don't be nervous – he will love it, and you can progress to holding him by the ankles and doing a gentle swing. Do this for as long as you can safely manage his weight. It is easier to roll him down on to his tummy, as he will arch his head backwards. You can then lift your baby by the arms so that he 'stands'.*

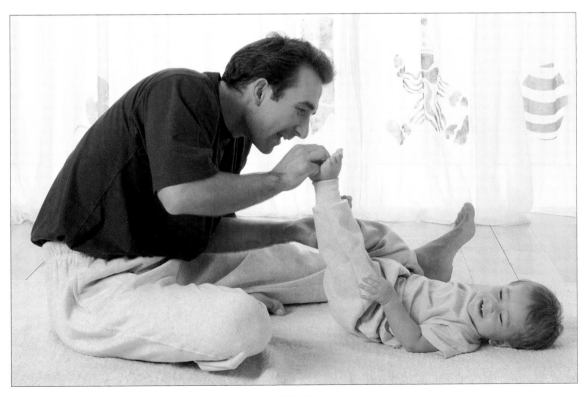

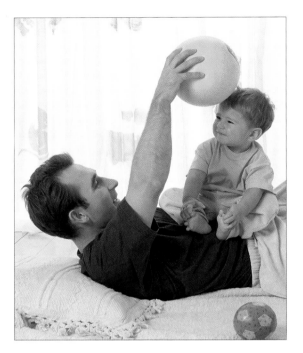

Make time for your baby to play, both alone and with you. Most babies make desperate attempts at this age to move from the spot. Objects fascinate, and encourage them to stretch out and grasp. Play with her across your knee, swinging her from side to side. Sing a rhythm, and hold her feet as she slides down onto the floor. She will, by twelve months, do a 'roll down' – tucking in her head. When you tire of this, she will still be saying 'again'.

Now your baby is one year old! A landmark. Why not celebrate with an aromatic massage and some musical fun (*see pages 48–50, 60 and 106*)?

Left and below. *Lie on the floor (safer than a bed) with your baby and make yourself comfortable with your head on a cushion. Let him crawl around you and over you, occasionally try to catch him between your legs or feet. He will love this and discover new games, too.*

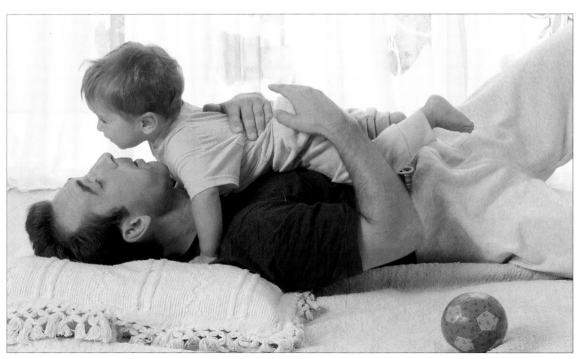

CHAPTER FIVE

On Their Own Two Feet

*I*t is just one year since you brought your baby into this world, and now it is impossible to imagine life without your child. You have both learned and seen and shared so much. All the signs of development into a child are now in place: talking, walking, playing, and relating to both parents as well as to others. As your child matures from one to two years old, both of you will sometimes be tested to the full. At fifteen months, she swings between reliance on an adult and independent action, sometimes rejecting the grown-ups' overtures. By twenty-one months she will briefly wait to be shown simple tasks.

At some time during the second year of your baby's life, you will see the first signs of the temper tantrums that are the hallmark of the Terrible Twos. Be prepared! This is the start of your child's free will emerging (see table on Temper Tantrums: How to Cope, on page 116).

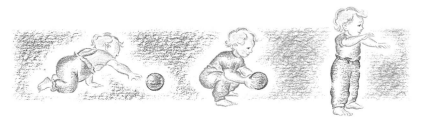

The Mobile Baby

By one year old, your baby is sitting unsupported for longer periods, crawling and often, by now, walking. Allow this process to develop naturally and assist your child only when she is ready to venture up on to her feet. Do not try to make her walk too soon as she will miss some of the crawling phase so vital to muscular and nervous-system coordination.

Between one and two years, your baby is active and noisy. She can crawl up and downstairs, is into cupboards and is curious about everything, still testing objects by putting them in her mouth. By two, she is surer on her feet and falls less often. She loves to climb on the furniture and may be a regular attender at Tumble Tots or Baby Gym classes.

She may have a vocabulary of around fifty words by the age of twenty months, the favourite of which seems to be 'NO'.

Parents sometimes feel that they need eyes in the back of their heads. Toddlers can move very quickly, but are as yet unaware of the hazards at home and outside.

Your toddler's routine may be settled, so that she eats and sleeps in regular patterns. Some babies this age still nap during the day.

Temper Tantrums: How to Cope

Therapy	What to do
Naturopathy	Eliminate anything salty, sugary or spicy from baby's diet, and from mother's if still breast-feeding
	Get out for long walks with baby as often as possible. Fresh air and a change of environment will help
	Keep baby to a regular sleep pattern
	Keep television watching to the minimum: passive entertainment increases boredom and frustration
Aromatherapy	Use 2 drops of essential oil – chamomile, neroli, lavender or mandarin – to 30ml almond carrier oil for delicious, soothing baby massage
	Use 1 drop neroli diluted in milk in baby's bathwater and allow plenty of time for a leisurely bath
	Put 1 drop neroli on cotton wool ball in baby's room before bedtime so that the same familiar smell greets her after bathtime
Bach flower remedies	Holly, aspen, vervain, impatiens or walnut
Herbalism	Chamomile, catnip, hops or limeflower drinks at bedtime
Homoeopathy	Consult your homoeopath
Colour therapy	Wear soft light colours, especially pale pink, and eliminate red as far as possible for the moment
Cranio-sacral	Consult your practitioner if baby's mood becomes overwhelming
Creative movement	Be supportive, not restrictive. Go with baby's mood. Choose favourite rhymes: play the music she likes

The Power of Touch

If you have been massaging your baby since she was tiny, by now you will have established what time of day is best, and the massage is usually completed in ten to fifteen minutes at most.

Starting to massage your child for the first time at this stage may be a little difficult, as young children do not want to keep still for long. But don't be deterred; your child will soon relish this close and loving contact.

A couple of drops of light citrus oils, such as mandarin, tangerine or orange, in 30ml of carrier oil are pleasant for young children. Among other essential oils, chamomile in particular is regarded as 'the children's oil' and 2 to 4 drops diluted in milk or vegetable oil can be added to the bath. Lavender, which has calming and soothing properties and helps promote sleep, can be used in the same way. If you wish to use either chamomile or lavender oil for baby massage, use 1 drop to 20ml of the carrier oil.

Yoga

From around sixteen months old, exercises can be extended into pre-yoga movements that will enhance your child's muscular flexibility. This is simply a matter of sitting on the floor with her and encouraging, not pushing or pulling, the child to stretch the body.

To start doing this, she may either (1) sit with the knees apart and the soles of the feet together (*see below*), or (2) she may be on her knees and sitting back with the toes pointing towards each other.

If she is in position (2), sit behind and encourage her to lean slowly back into your lap; in this way she will be exercising her legs and back.

Left. *Most toddlers sit with perfect posture. The head is held up and the shoulders relaxed.*

Below. *It only takes a little coaxing to get your child to lean forward, the soles of the feet together. Starting from here she can work towards getting her head on the floor.*

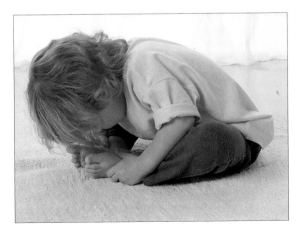

From One to Two Years: The Herbal Options

Condition	What to Use
Restless or impatient	Bach flower remedies: impatiens, holly, walnut
Teething	Let baby chew on marshmallow stick or licorice stick. Rub gums with glycerine or honey. Give infusions of either chamomile, limeflower, yarrow, fennel or catnip regularly through the day
Insomnia, hyperactivity	Infusions of chamomile, catnip, hops or limeflower
	Bach flower remedies: vervain, impatiens, holly, aspen or walnut
Low mood	Bach flower remedies: walnut, aspen, mimulus or Star of Bethlehem
Cuts and grazes	Bach flower remedies: Star of Bethlehem or Rescue Remedy
Jealousy and sibling rivalry	Bach flower remedies: holly, aspen or walnut. Chamomile, catnip herbal infusions
Nightmares	Bach flower remedies: aspen or mimulus
Needing independence	Bach flower remedy: walnut

Your Baby's Perception

Sight involves the perception of colour, form, depth and movement. From the age of one year, the infant's interest in strong, bright colours grows. Children show a marked preference for the colour red. This is because red is a colour which helps the incarnated soul to become integrated into the earth planet, a process which continues up until puberty.

The aura or electromagnetic field that surrounds children is also becoming stronger and, as well as red, both orange and yellow take on greater depth. Up to the age of five, an infant is able to see auras and can easily detect from them people's moods and well-being. A wonderful story is told of a five year old who opened the front door for a visitor and then ran back to his mother to announce that there was a man on the doorstep wearing a red suit. When the mother went to investigate, she found a very angry man wearing a grey suit. What the child had seen was the man's aura, which was red with anger. If a child is born into a family who follow and are well versed in esotericism, it is possible to keep a child's auric sight open. If not, then by the age of seven this gift will have closed down.

From approximately eighteen months, the infant has a fascination for putting containers inside each other and for sorting out building bricks by colour and size. This is an age when the child can discover a great deal through colour. She can learn not only the size of containers and bricks by their colour but also many other skills. A child's brain, like an adult's, contains a left and right hemisphere. The left hemisphere works with the intellect, whereas the right hemisphere works with both the intuition and creativity. Playing with coloured containers and bricks works with both hemispheres, thereby bringing them into balance. The shape of the bricks/containers works with the left hemisphere and the colour works with the right hemisphere.

Experiments carried out with mentally impaired children have shown that they will remember which coat and hat belongs to them by the colour of the peg that these are hung on. It has been found that colour plays an important role in teaching such children.

In order to enhance and encourage the four elements of sight:
• Extend and introduce more complicated and coordinated games.
• Give your child good models to imitate.
• Develop catching and throwing games.
• Give your child the palming exercise when telling her a story.
• Maintain active listening to support your baby's emotional development.
• Allow your child to express feelings freely, within given boundaries; this can help reduce parental fatigue.
• Avoid imposing meaningless polite behaviour, which distorts the child's healthy emotional development and induces only tension and fatigue in you.
• Play 'no!' games.

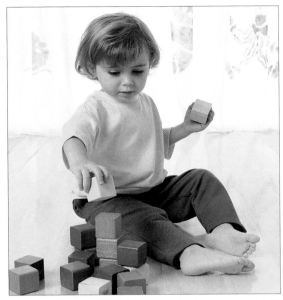

Above. *Playing with bricks helps develop the use of right and left brains with binocular focusing.*

• Provide paper, pencils, felt tips, crayons and plasticine for your baby to play with (check before buying that they are safe for baby and toddler use).
• Play with speech and sound.
• Go over the exercises given previously, in Chapter Two (*see pages 83–4*), in Chapter Three (*see pages 97–8*), and in Chapter Four (*see page 109*).

Your Baby's Structure

If until now the physical structure has been balanced out, your baby should be well established with normal healthy growth and function. But a child's body is growing every day. Any development imprinted on it by illness or injuries can set up an inappropriate pattern of growth which should be treated by an osteopath before it becomes permanent. Spinal curvatures can appear apparently out of the blue. Falls and knocks can leave restrictions and asymmetries in the spine or pelvis as a focus for aberrant growth. Infectious diseases, tummy bugs and all sorts of illnesses can create a focus of irritation not only in individual organs but also reflecting out into the general structure. These may particularly affect the spine, creating areas of tension and therefore restricted mobility, with effects on the

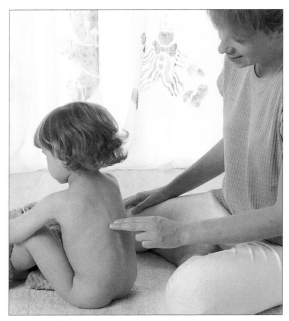

Above. *When you run your fingers down your baby's spine, you may find areas of restriction reflecting internal disorders. If so consult an osteopath promptly.*

overall structural balance and posture. These exert strains on the back, pelvis and neck and consequently the internal organs can function less efficiently.

If you examine your baby's spine by touch, this can sometimes reveal areas of tightness caused by untoward tensions. It is always best in this case to lose no time in seeking the advice of an osteopath.

Osteopathy can be used throughout childhood to iron out any asymmetries and to deal with the effects of accidents and illnesses. It can also be used to mobilize and release the abdomen, pelvis and thorax. This can have the effect of treating digestive disturbances and protecting against asthma and other respiratory conditions. It can be used to treat infectious conditions directly, by means of lymphatic drainage work.

The Cranio-sacral Check

Any slowness in your baby's physical or mental development is best referred to a cranio-sacral therapist. Indications of poor coordination or slow development of speech may be due to cranial bone restrictions, or other constrictions within the cranio-sacral system.

As your baby begins to walk, she is likely to fall over frequently, and repeatedly bang her head, so a cranio-sacral check-up is still advisable every three months or so.

This is especially so after any severe fall, illness or shock, particularly if it appears to leave your child adversely affected, physically or emotionally; also if such disorders as headache, digestive ailment, irritability, restlessness or moodiness seem to persist.

Tantrums and behavioural difficulties are common at this age and may just be normal. However, tantrums can be brought on by accidents, especially a head injury or emotional shock. So, if the change of behaviour follows some incident, the child should be checked to see if there are physical effects within the cranio-sacral system.

If her tempestuous behaviour has been developing since an early age and is now simply aggravated, there may be some underlying cause. This too may be something which a skilled cranio-sacral therapist could resolve.

The struggle for mobility throughout your child's second year is bound to bring bumps and bruises. By her first birthday she can walk with one hand held; a year later she will be able to go up and down stairs unaided. In between, she will learn feats that include standing up unsupported, running, throwing a ball without falling, and walking alone with a gait which is no longer broad-based or high-stepping.

Such triumphs are rarely achieved without mishaps, some of which may well call for investigation by a therapist.

Your Baby's Playtime

This is high-risk time for exasperation and accidents! Because babies are now usually walking, running, breaking things and having minor accidents, they can seem physically ahead of their sense of space and distance.

The more practice they have had in running around, managing themselves and learning about gravity and dynamics, the more skilled they are in avoiding endless bumps and bruises. They will be far safer and less prone to frustrations and tantrums.

One to two year olds need time and space in which to move and play, more than any other age group. Their bodies will be stronger and their backs straighter than before. Their energy can seem terrifying – but what's the use of new strong legs and buttocks if you can't use them? Try to remember that some nearly two year olds can be very timid and find their 'friends' hard to cope with. It is vital for these children to have scope in which to grow more confident through movement, so that they can learn relating to others through play.

By this time you can follow the class idea in Chapter One (*see pages 60–65*). Make sure you clear a space – two year olds crashing around can cause damage. Try to go along with the children's energy and avoid head-on confrontation if you can. Leave plenty of time for their ideas and don't expect instant cooperation in sharing. Their newly acquired sense of self makes giving things up painful. They scream 'mine' constantly. You can practise 'giving' games such as handing over a toy on your request. Sometimes they tremble with the agony and need huge reassurance and praise.

Find time to dance together. Put on some music and bop. On every possible occasion encourage them to run, skip, balance, and find things to climb.

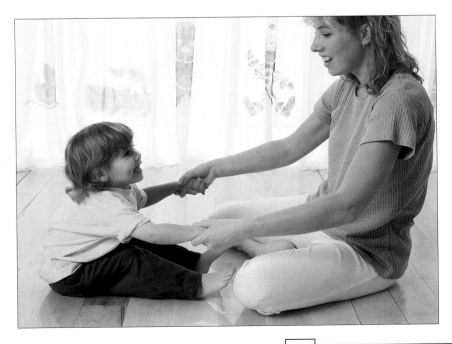

Left. *Two year olds can be on the receiving end of a constant stream of instructions – 'Be careful.' 'Don't touch.' 'Hurry up.' 'Not so noisy, please.' Take time to sit down together, hold hands, talk, and share a few quiet moments. Decide what you want to do and prepare to practise some strength skills. Remember that being strong is a new and exciting idea for children of this age. Play the game of I can lift / carry / push / pull / squeeze. Try it with a cushion.*

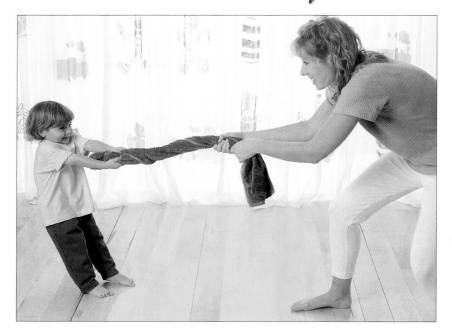

Left. *There are lots of games you and your child can play with a towel. Roll it up and tug it, or thump it against the floor. Alternatively, at bathtime, catch her, wrap her up and dry her, all in play. Try the game of 'push me over', either standing firm or crouched over your knees. Tell her, 'Hold on to my back and I'll shake you off – hold tight.' 'Push your feet/hands against mine. I'll hold you tight and see if you can get away.' She will respond with shrieks of delight.*

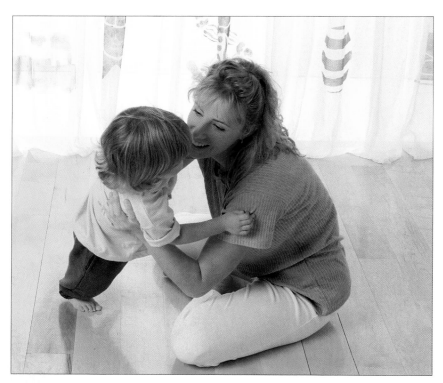

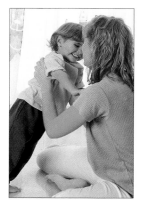

Left and above. *Wrestling. Most children adore mock fights. Hold your child under the arms and ask her to place her hands on your shoulders. Say 'Ready – now push – heave ho.' Someone (usually you) will end up on the floor.*

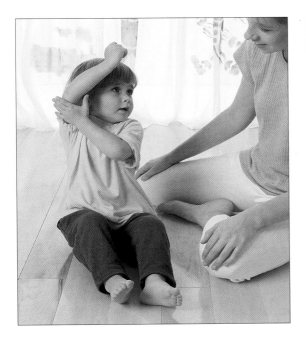

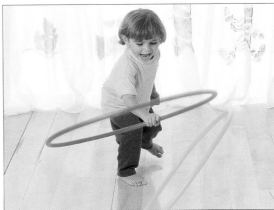

Above. *Learning to 'work' a toy, such as a hoop, makes for a wider and bolder range of movements.*

Left. *Mobility. Children love body parts at this age. You can introduce joints, asking them, 'Wiggle your fingers, circle your ankles. What does your elbow do? Your knee?'*

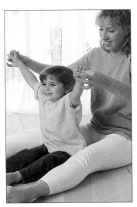

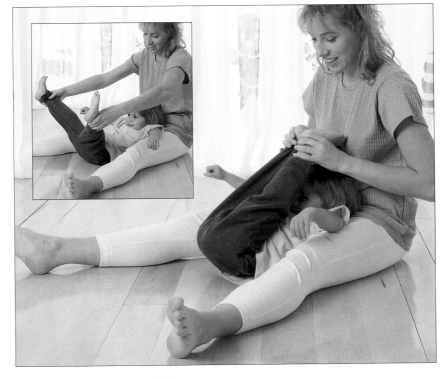

Above, right and inset. *Stretches. Being more flexible than most adults, your child will probably find it fun to copy simple stretches. Ask her, 'Stretch out like a star – can you miaow and stretch like a cat? Can you catch your feet?'*

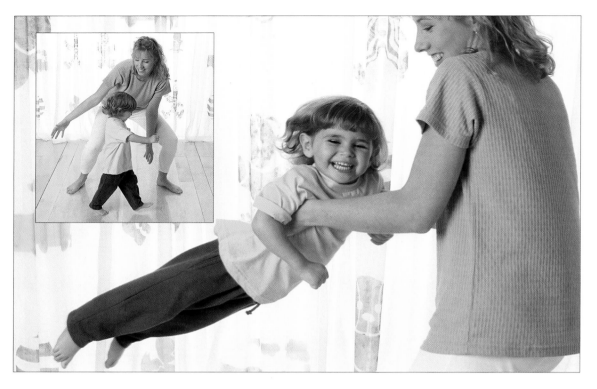

Above. *Agility is the main pleasure of childhood. Children love combinations of movements: running and jumping; walking and turning; being lifted and swung. The confidence these bring is crucial to growing up.*

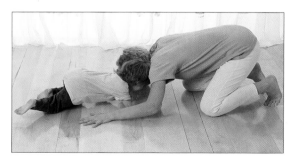

Above. *Try crawling along on all fours, imitating snakes and crocodiles, and playing at going to sleep. This is the beginning of 'Let's pretend.' Your child's desire for play may now include many simple games of make-believe which she will want to share with an adult.*

If crawling and walking were the previous preoccupations, now it is climbing. Allow time to explore the spaces at home. Make clear that climbing on chairs, beds and sofas must not be done alone. Point out that falling and hitting the floor will hurt.

Set aside an old armchair for practising – your child can try to heave herself onto it, slide down, move the cushion, jump off, crawl across, balance, ride astride the back, and bounce on it. Let her do just as she wishes, during this important time for releasing energy.

Now your baby has reached the age of two and it is time to move on in emotional and developmental terms. She is more a young child than a little baby and there will be marvellous new opportunities in which parents can relish their child's company, personality, and interesting quirks of behaviour.

CHAPTER SIX

The Human Dynamo

The 'Terrible Twos' is characterized by tantrums and at about two and a half by negativism, manifesting itself as a refusal to do anything the child's mother wants, whether bathing, sleeping, getting dressed or going for a walk. However, this stage does not last long and the positive outlook of the three year old child more than makes up for it.

The two year old will typically be a mass of contradictions in that she is fiercely independent but clingy, rebellious yet attention-seeking. Some people regard this age of child as the most attractive, on account of its charm and liveliness and an absence of the fully fledged stubbornness and aggressive behaviour so often seen in older children.

This is the time to expose your child to as many new experiences as you can, for she has reached a point at which her energy and curiosity know no bounds.

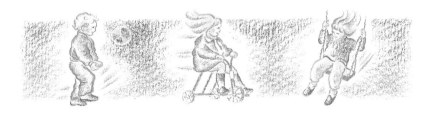

Your Child's New Achievements

At two years old your child will be able to walk up and down the stairs while carrying something, and will play happily for short periods alone, performing quite complicated roles such as undressing a doll, putting it to bed and reading it a story.

She will have a full set of milk teeth by the time she is two and a half and will be quite physically strong – enough to kick a ball and move large toys around. Scribbling will give way to more recognizable drawing and she will be able to paint with a large brush. Make sure that she has all the crayons, paper, paint and brushes that she needs at this important stage of development.

Continue developing her musical ear by playing your child lots of different types of music. You can take out cassette tapes and compact discs from your local library. Make sure that your child has several simple musical instruments through which she can express musical energy and rhythm.

No longer a toddler, your two year old is now an energetic, demanding little person: a human dynamo. She has gained control over bowels and bladder during the day and is rapidly building up a vocabulary. She loves to run and climb and explore, and is rarely still for a minute. She demands a great deal of attention and makes a fuss and throws tantrums if frustrated. As she begins to assert independence, she can appear to be very rebellious and stubborn. This age of childhood is, in fact, entirely self-centred.

If it all becomes too much for either parent, look back to Aromatic Solutions in earlier chapters for a choice of refreshing and invigorating oils. Use these in massage or in a vaporizer; in particular, try essential oils of lemon, geranium or rosemary.

By three years old your baby is now very grown up, and much more sociable and willing and eager to play and mix with other children. She is more confident if neither parent is around for a while, and usually very agile and much more coordinated in movement.

Children still need quiet play and restful calm periods to relax in. Constant activity and stimulation can lead to irritability and over-tiredness. A two to three year old has a tremendous resistance to sleep and will very rarely be napping any longer during the day. At this age they seem to think or know that they are going to miss something interesting as soon as they have fallen asleep and cannot bear to have to go off to bed. Sleeplessness (and resistance to potty training) can be treated effectively by your homoeopath.

Foundation for the Future

Children today are growing up taller and heavier, and physically doing much less, than they were twenty-five years ago.

In Britain, a national survey of diet and nutrition published in March 1995 found that 75 per cent of children aged between one and a half and four and a half consumed large quantities of biscuits, white bread, sugary drinks, chips and sweets; 43 per cent ate sugary sweets; and 24 per cent consumed fizzy drinks nearly every day. On the other hand, the same survey found that raw vegetables and salad were included in their diet by less than 25 per cent of children in the same age group; and only 39 per cent were in the habit of eating green vegetables.

Now is the time to educate your child's palate for life. Make sure her diet includes adequate quantities of green leafy vegetables, salads, fruit, fish, cheese and eggs, and wholemeal (rather than white) products. Your child should be eating plenty of wholemeal bread and well-soaked muesli-type cereals in favour of over-processed, sugary and salty foods.

Only in this way will she receive the nutrients she needs for the formation of strong bones and a healthy body. A good diet provides the child with the energy she needs for a full and active day, without resorting to sweets for a swift lift. Good, regular exercise is also essential to your child's healthy development, including the establishment of a strong immune system.

Many of the common complaints and disorders suffered by children in their very early years have been discussed in earlier chapters. How to deal with temper tantrums, a feature of the Terrible Twos, has been described in the previous chapter (*see page 116*), as this period often starts before the child actually reaches her birthday. (*For other complaints, consult the A–Z in Part Three, pages 135–56.*)

It is timely now to turn back to Part One and reread the individual therapies, to see how best each therapy may be applied to your child now that you know her so much better.

The Power of Touch

Bathtime or just before bed may be the favoured time for massage if your child has been receiving this since babyhood.

It is not so easy, though, to begin massage for the first time on a toddler, as they usually want to run off and do something else. Nonetheless, it is worth a try, so if you are only just starting to massage your child it is probably a good idea to begin with just the legs and feet the first time. Maybe the back can be massaged the second time, and the belly and arms and hands the third time. Probably you will have your child's attention and interest while doing just a part of the massage. You can bring all the parts together when the time is right.

Often between the ages of two and three your child, now so much more active, may want to give you a massage back, partly because she wants to get hold of the oil and rub it everywhere!

It is nice to encourage your child by just letting her massage your feet, or your hands or face and head. Some children seem to know instinctively how to massage. Try letting her massage your scalp with the fingertips, ideally in deep circular movements. It feels wonderful.

Aromatherapy for the Two Year Old

Condition	Essential Oil	How to Use
Sleeplessness	2 drops chamomile	In your child's bathwater (diluted in milk)
Fretting	2 drops chamomile	In your child's bathwater (diluted in milk)
Frustration, tantrums	2 drops of chamomile, neroli, lavender or mandarin	On a cotton wool ball in your child's room
(*See Chapter Five, page 116*)	2 drops of chamomile, neroli, lavender or mandarin	In 30ml almond oil, as a foot massage

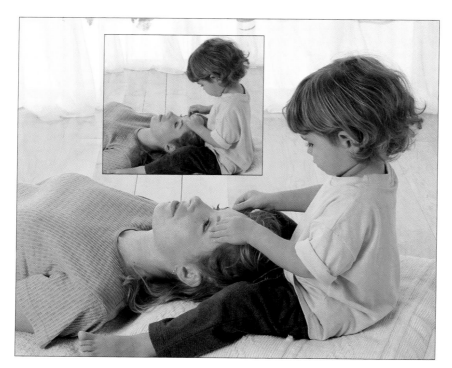

Left, inset. *If you lie down on the floor and your child sits at your head, she can give you a face massage. Show her how to stroke the fingertips across your forehead. You can take her hands and guide them across, giving hints about pressure. Just slide them across from the centre of your forehead out to your temples.*

Left. *Stroke her hands gently over your eyelids. Come back to the cheeks and stroke across your cheekbones towards the ears, following the shape of the bones.*

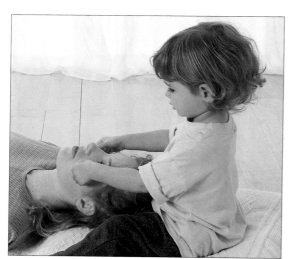

Above. *Circle your child's fingertips into your cheeks. Explain to her how she can stroke across the area between your nose and top lip out to the corner of your mouth. Then have her stroke under your lower lip to the corner of your mouth.*

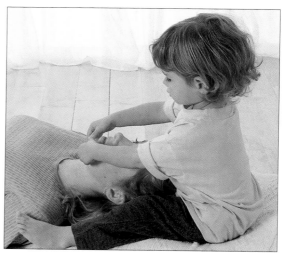

Above. *Show her how to work along your chin, squeezing the jawbone between the thumbs and forefingers, and out to the ears. You will soon discover that having your ears massaged between the thumb and forefinger feels lovely too!*

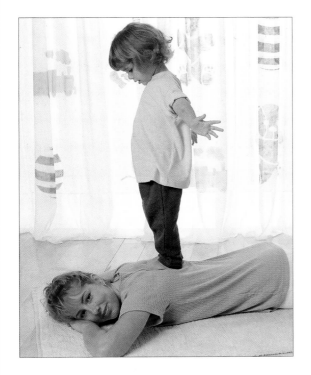

Your three year old can be quite therapeutic for a tired aching back, too. She is just the right weight now to be able to walk on you. Ask your partner or a friend to help the first couple of times. Lie face down on the floor (you don't need to remove any clothes), with your child barefoot. She might need some help to get her balance at first and she needs to feel for the right place to step, so the first couple of times might be a bit hit and miss.

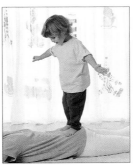

Left and far left. *Your child can step sideways along your back so that she can slide step from your shoulders down to your sacrum and back again. Alternatively, she can stand facing along your body and have one foot either side of your spine.*

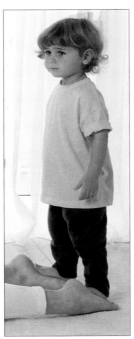

Right. *Have your bare feet relaxed with the toes pointing comfortably towards each other. Next, you should persuade your child to place her feet over your insteps. She does need to be able to balance fairly well here, in order that she can remain upright. Then have your child 'walk' her feet on the spot, all the while shifting her body weight from foot to foot. She can also do this with her back to you, so that she is stepping on to the soles of your feet with her heels over your instep, and thereby 'walking'.*

After your have shown your child how to do it a couple of times, she will soon be doing it for you without your help. Now you can truly say your child 'walks all over you' and mean something entirely pleasurable!

The Cranio-sacral Check

Treatment of your child at this age can be divided into two main categories:

1 Good cranio-sacral treatment from an early age should have helped to make her healthy and happy, and less likely to need further treatment. A check-up every six months, or whenever there is cause for concern, should suffice.

2 Children who have not been treated earlier may need more regular attention now, in order to deal with problems which may otherwise become more ingrained.

Various illnesses and injuries will occur at this age, as throughout childhood and adult life, which may be amenable to cranio-sacral treatment. By now, though, the emphasis will ideally have shifted away from treating conditions and disorders towards maintaining good health. Just as regular visits to the dentist are likely to ensure strong teeth, so regular visits to the cranio-sacral therapist will help to produce a healthy, happy child.

If each incident is treated and resolved as it occurs throughout childhood, this sets the pattern for the future, through not allowing apparently minor injuries to affect patterns of growth and development and thereby causing problems later in life.

Your Child's Perception

During the ages of two to three years, the use of colour in all of life is important: in toys, the child's surroundings and the clothes that she wears. Try allowing her to choose the colours she wears. A child is extremely sensitive to the vibrations of colour and will, in all probability, choose the colours that she needs. If you have a garden which is safe to play in, allow this as often as possible. The colours of nature are 'living' ones and extremely beneficial both mentally and physically.

Colours that are important at this age are red, orange, yellow and blue. Red, an 'earthing' colour, is also the colour of energy, warmth and vitality. Orange is a colour of joy and creativity and helps in exploring the wonders of life. It also assists the powers of expression that enable this. Yellow is a bright sunny colour, which makes it attractive to many young children. It is also the colour that stimulates the child's fast-developing brain. Blue, as already mentioned, is the colour of peace, rest and tranquillity. This makes it excellent for a child who is over-active or over-tired and refuses to sleep.

Through working with colour together with your child, you will discover for yourself its vibrant and healing world. Remembering that perception and vision rests on colour, form, movement and depth, put into practice some of the teachings of the Bates method.

Bates Method

• Help your child to play act. Encourage pretend and dressing-up games.
• Help your child to play with tongue twisters, hide-and-seek and 'looking for' games.
• Play balancing games.
• Do your best to be interested in your child's what? and why? questions. These are often profound with no easy answer. It is destructive to the child's development to ignore such questions as they are an important key to active seeing and active focusing in the mind. It is better to admit ignorance if necessary and to look for the answers together.

These questions often show a clear window on life in contrast to the adult world of pretence and subterfuge.
• Allow your child to express an independent will – within acceptable boundaries – so helping the growth of confidence.
• Give opportunities for vigorous play.
• Avoiding expectations and demands can help parents adjust to the human dynamo.
• When the question of pre-school arises, debate its value and for whose benefit it is being proposed. Is your child ready for an early exile?

Avoid dogmatic attitudes to this and to premature pressure to achieve. It is often more useful to see what a particular child's needs are in order to help her find her own pace.

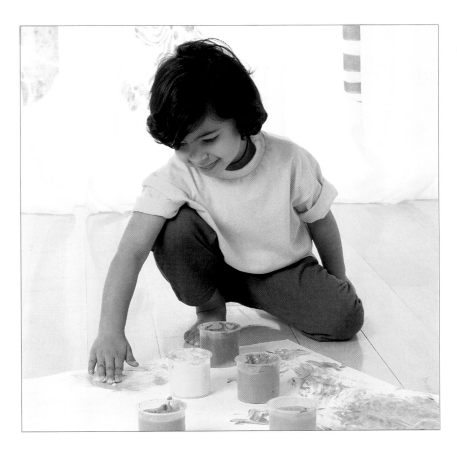

Left. *At two and three years old, a child loves to use crayons and paints. Her pictures may seem to an adult nothing more than scribble, but to her they are symbolic. Through the medium of colour, children are interpreting their world and the people that surround them. Try asking your child to explain her painting and to say why she chose certain colours.*

Your Child's Playtime

The tempestuous twos often settle down as speech and vocabulary develop and they gain confidence from growing more physically skilled and socially adept.

They adore their playtime classes and will remind you exactly how to begin. By now they can be quite bossy and organized, and will copy and mimic everyone, especially the family. They love dressing up (have a bag of old hats, scarves etc.); and all sorts of fantasy play, such as tea parties, shops, school, building houses with chairs and blankets, and dollies and bicycles. They have jokes and songs and stories and are much more biddable.

Children who have practised creative movement are by now very skilled and agile movers with an excellent sense of space and distance. Keep the old armchair for tumble play. It will now be a ship, shop or car which helps them enjoy long periods of fantasy play – 'Let's pretend we're on a boat.' They love stunts: head over heels on the chair, shouting 'one-two-three go' and balancing and jumping off, standing astride the seat, then bouncing and sliding head first on to the floor.

They love to share ideas with you: 'Watch me – can you do it too?' They enjoy new tricks: 'Show me how to do a cartwheel.' 'Hold my feet and I'll do a handstand.' (Be careful to support their backs.) Head-over-heels in sequences is usually popular, too. They will love to do stunts with you. This is important play. It gives children a real thrill and is a physical discipline and challenge. It is fun for the adult to take part, too.

Lie on the floor, knees bent and let your child sit on your knees. Hold her feet up and arms out like a statue.

Have your child stand up tall like a candle. Lie her on her tummy along your shins to imitate a flying bird.

Your child will play tag (but at three she will probably still like to chase and not be chased) and any simple games such as hide and seek and 'What's the time Mr Wolf?' (probably hiding only her eyes), but never for long. She will decide when to change games.

Do not attempt to compete with your child. Three year olds rarely play in order to win; at this age the keyword is cooperation.

Organize simple group games. Three year olds love to hold hands in a circle and skip. Change direction and combine with clapping – they can even do the 'hokey-cokey' and musical bumps provided that everyone 'wins'.

They will be adept at building 'the track', pushing chairs around and making piles of cushions here and there, and will tell you how it works. They will be cautious and clever, knowing exactly if they can fit into a space without bumping heads. 'You're too big to get under there,' they will say.

They love inventing new games and have a great pride in what they can manage to do. By four, there will be shouts of 'easy peasy' if things are not challenging enough, but at two and three they glow with pride and often repeat the same pattern over and over again. Some children have an instinctive ability to manage a ball, while others show less interest.

They will possibly never have excellent hand-eye coordination, but they may be very skilled in playing with plastic hoops, rope, skittles, or bean bags, for example.

A large ball is the easiest to manage at this age and the skills of rolling, throwing, kicking, bouncing and catching are quickly achieved. Your child will be learning to count and there will be much 'One – two – three – four – I did five that time!'

Introduce any new toy carefully. Give your child plenty of time to explore it. 'Have you seen this before?' She will be learning to look at things carefully and be very creative with her play now. Show one new toy at a time rather than a pile, which she will discard almost immediately.

Give your child tasks which she has to perform tidily and concentrate on and remember, matching words with actions: 'Pick up the cushion – run to the corner – put it on the floor and sit on it.' Another matching game is: 'Run to the gate and then walk back on your hands and feet like a camel while I count to see how long you take.' 'Walk round the table, clap three times and hop on one foot.' The ideas are endless. Don't make them too difficult, though. Insist on care and neatness. She may think up some tasks for you to try, too.

There must be time for social games, such as pouring imaginary tea, playing at cooking or pretending that she is mummy, daddy or the new baby.

Children often do their class with a doll or teddy as companion: 'I'm giving my baby a dance about.' They play out their fears and anxieties ('Teddy's going to see the doctor'), and become more confident and therefore more secure in their surroundings. In this way they learn to relate more easily to others, are never bored and are more apt to be physically fit, strong and skilled.

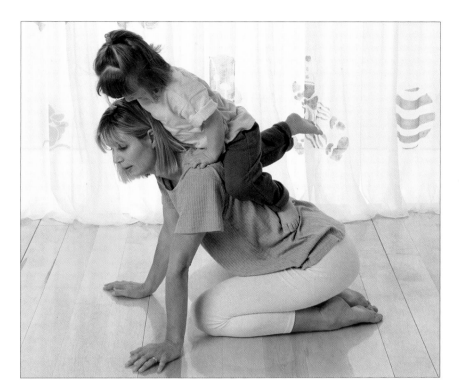

Left. *By the time they are three, children will think of their own tricks such as sitting, and then standing up, on your shoulders. Avoid falls and don't attempt anything which might alarm your child. She will not be critical of you, of course, but convinced that your joint efforts are perfect.*

Below. *Your child will now enjoy long inventive games, for example trying to return the treat of being pulled around on a cushion. She is discovering the limits of her strength and solving its problems: 'Push with your feet.'*

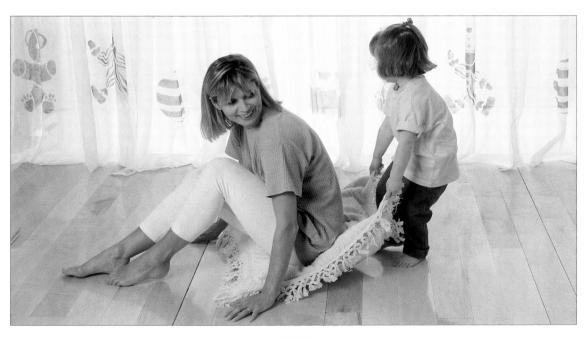

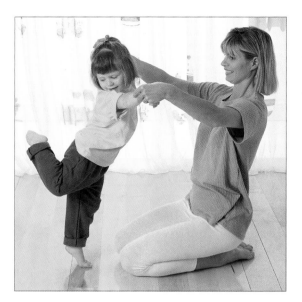

Left. *Miraculously, your child will be able to spring and jump now and will prance and skip and jump endlessly. Encourage her by holding her hands and skipping, too: 'We'll dance together.' Try asking: 'Can you hop on one foot?' 'Can you gallop sideways?'*

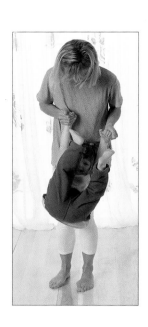

Right. *She will be much stronger now, so much so that she is able to lift up her legs as she tries to turn upside down.*

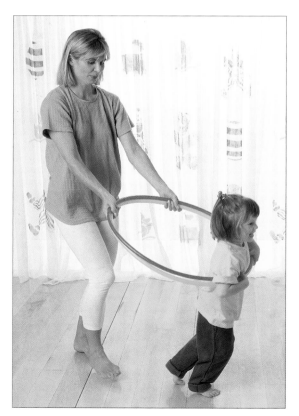

Left. *Try playing with hoops together. 'It's called a hoop – feel it – it's made of plastic – what colour is it? – Green – like the grass – it's light – and it's smooth – what shape is it? – That's right – it's a circle.' Share your experience with your child: 'Can you climb through it? Put it over your head? Roll it, spin it, put it down flat and jump into it? Play horse and cart – I'll be the horse.'*

Movement play is not an optional extra to be fitted in as and when there is time. It is the natural way of life for a child. Playing and moving together gives both parents and child a new understanding and enjoyment of everything about one another.

These suggestions are only starting points. Allow the child's own pace and favourite interests to provide the lead. Use the play movement themes to increase your own skills, too.

Your child is now three: light years in developmental and emotional terms from the helpless baby you gave birth to just a short while ago. Keep her with you in the natural way as much as you can. Above all, enjoy your child to the full. Childhood is short.

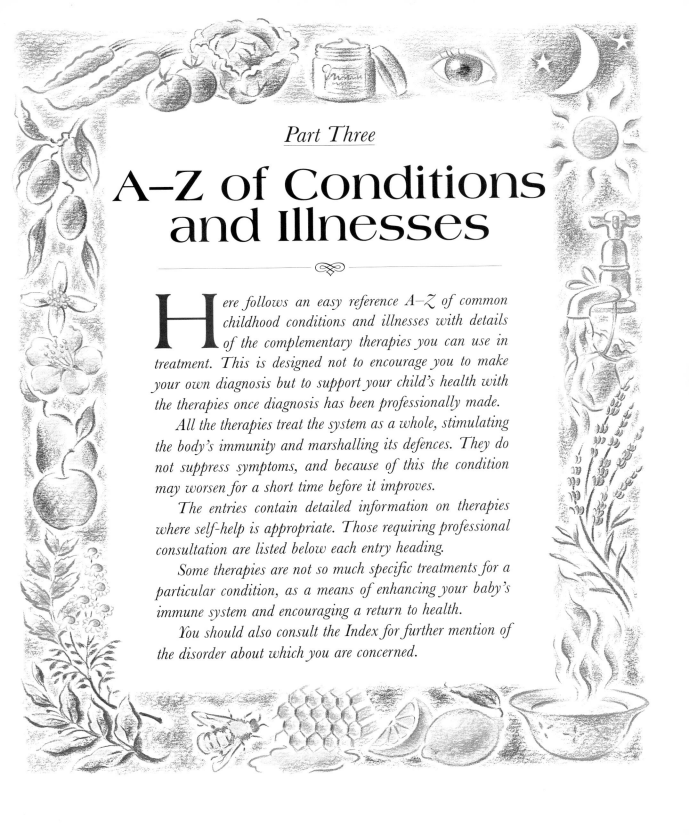

Part Three

A–Z of Conditions and Illnesses

❧

Here follows an easy reference A–Z of common childhood conditions and illnesses with details of the complementary therapies you can use in treatment. This is designed not to encourage you to make your own diagnosis but to support your child's health with the therapies once diagnosis has been professionally made.

All the therapies treat the system as a whole, stimulating the body's immunity and marshalling its defences. They do not suppress symptoms, and because of this the condition may worsen for a short time before it improves.

The entries contain detailed information on therapies where self-help is appropriate. Those requiring professional consultation are listed below each entry heading.

Some therapies are not so much specific treatments for a particular condition, as a means of enhancing your baby's immune system and encouraging a return to health.

You should also consult the Index for further mention of the disorder about which you are concerned.

In an Emergency

Seek professional medical treatment without delay if your child has any of the following:

• breathlessness or difficulty in breathing • unexplained, abnormal drowsiness
• fever of 101° F (38.5° C) or more • convulsions (fits) • severe headache • impaired vision,
especially with headache • any severe pain or obvious distress • much vomiting, diarrhoea or
constipation • stiff neck, particularly combined with dislike of bright light • refusing food

Allergies

True allergies are not as common as supposed. The typical reaction swiftly follows exposure to the offending substance and symptoms are usually a wheeze, watery nasal or eye discharge, a skin rash, or diarrhoea. More common are intolerances to some foods which, if incompletely digested, may create symptoms without involvement of the immune system.

• Aromatherapy
• Homoeopathy
• Kinesiology
• Osteopathy
• Cranio-sacral
  therapy

Naturopathy If your child has a true allergy it is sensible to avoid exposure to the triggering factors, such as cow's milk or animal fur, but more important to reduce susceptibility. Acute allergic reactions may be relieved by a short programme of juices and vegetables only. Carrot, apple, and cucumber juices or pineapple, apple, and parsley juices are good combinations which may be given for 24 or 48 hours. To reduce susceptibility exclude all sweet foods for some weeks.

A naturopath may prescribe physiologically balanced mineral supplements or other constitutional remedies to assist healing.

BIOCHEMIC TISSUE SALTS FOR ALLERGIES

Remedy	Dose
Natrum mur	3 cellules every two hours for watery discharges
Natrum sulph	3 cellules every two hours for stuffy congestive conditions
Ferrum phos	3 cellules every one to two hours for acute and irritative conditions

Herbalism Give evening primrose oil or borage seed oil to provide gamma linoleic acid, for normal functioning of the immune system.

Borage, chamomile, cinnamon, echinacea, lemon balm, yarrow, licorice, and red clover can be used singly or in combination to build resistance to allergies.

Give chamomile and yarrow tea daily to inhibit the production of histamine, responsible for many inflammatory symptoms. Nettles, in tea, soups and stews, also calm the allergic response. Herbs for the liver may be added to the prescriptions, for example, dandelion leaf, yellow dock or rosemary.

Allergies
(cont.)

Anxiety
• Colour therapy
• Osteopathy
• Cranio-sacral
  therapy

Bates method This may help alleviate such eye conditions as itching, puffiness, watering, strain and ache. Try palming; covering the closed eyes with moist lint, alternately warm and cool, always within the comfort zone; gently running a finger in an infinity sign around the orbits of the eyes; looking at a green colour. Also try a few drops of witch hazel lotion or calendula tincture in the water moistening the lint.

Massage This condition often responds well to massage.

Aromatherapy For nightmares: chamomile baths with 1–2 drops diluted in milk, or 1–2 drops on a cotton wool ball in child's room to calm her.

Herbalism Vervain, skullcap and wild oats strengthen the nervous system, and can make the child less vulnerable to tension. Oats are tonic for the nervous system, given in decoction or in porridge, muesli or flapjacks. Chamomile, limeflower and catmint are relaxing. Cinnamon, licorice and borage will increase resistance to stress and the latter two act as tonics to the adrenal glands. Liver remedies such as dandelion root, vervain or rosemary should be added to the prescription.

Bach flower remedies Aspen, mimulus, white chestnut or rock rose can be given four times daily, or more if necessary.

HOMOEOPATHY FOR ANXIETY	
Details of Condition	**Remedy**
Sudden anxiety with fear; this may follow an accident	Aconite
Anxiety about health; fastidiousness; liking company; anxiety about dying; restlessness and chilliness	Arsenicum album
Anxiety before performing in public – even at playgroup	Gelsemium
Anxiety about the dark as night falls; needs company; extreme fear of ghosts and being alone; thirst for cold drinks	Phosphorous

Bates method It is important that the child is willing to receive help. Is the mother herself transferring anxiety? Palming may help; also most of the procedures in Part Two (*see pages 83–4, 97–8, 109, 119 and 130*).

Kinesiology As for allergies, except it is an active awareness of the anxiety which is held in the energy field during the balancing procedure. Try touching the ESR points while the baby is distressed.

Movement and dance Creative movement can also relieve anxiety.

Asthma

Asthma is often the consequence of an allergic reaction, so general recommendations for dealing with allergies may be followed. It often occurs in association with eczema (see separate entry), especially if the latter has been suppressed with creams. Infantile eczema treated in this way may often result in asthma developing after two or three years as the hypersensitivity of the skin is driven deeper to the mucous membranes of the lungs. During an acute attack always seek medical help as this can be life-saving.

- Homoeopathy
- Colour therapy
- Bates method
- Osteopathy
- Cranio-sacral therapy
- Alexander technique

Naturopathy For wheezing, use the mild detoxification programme (*see page 12*) to relieve the burden on skin and lungs. Reduce mucus-forming foods such as cow's-milk products, sugar, and other refined carbohydrates. Increase leafy vegetables and carrots for protective nutrients, and seeds and seed oils or tahini for essential fatty acids. Older children may have warm compresses to relieve constriction of the airways.

BIOCHEMIC TISSUE SALTS FOR ASTHMA	
Remedy	How to Use
Kali phos	3 cellules every half to one hour for wheezy, tight or oppressed breathing and nervous asthma
Natrum mur	3 cellules every one to two hours for wheezy chest with productive cough

Massage Most effective is the cupping technique over the back. Lay the child on her front across your lap with her head tipped lower than the body. Tap her back and sides with your hands in a cupped position. This should set up a slight vibration in the chest which will help loosen mucus. Your baby might cough as the mucus comes up. Regular should allow relaxed breathing using the diaphragm and lungs fully.

Aromatherapy Regular back massage, using gentle essential oils such as lavender, neroli and chamomile, can be of enormous help. These are anti-spasmodic and anti-depressant, and can relieve spasm and the stress trigger. It is vital to consult an holistic aromatherapist, as some asthmatics react to perfumes and essential oils.

Herbalism Herbs may need to be given over a few months, sometimes with inhalers or other medication from the doctor. These may be gradually reduced as the condition improves.

For the immune system, borage, chamomile, garlic and licorice can be combined with other herbs to relax the bronchi and expel mucus. These include coltsfoot, lungwort, mullein, thyme or elecampane.

Add herbs to relieve irritation of the bronchi leading to constriction; for example, marshmallow, slippery elm, lungwort, mullein or plantain.

Licorice has expectorant properties and supports the adrenal glands, providing a natural counterpart to cortisone and reducing stress and the allergic response. This is an advantage for children using cortisone inhalers or internal medication, for which you may want alternatives. Herbs that support the nervous system and counter tension can be

Asthma
(cont.)

added. These include chamomile, limeflower, skullcap or vervain. During an attack, hot foot-baths can be made using the same herbs for infusions. Hot compresses of these can be applied frequently to the chest. Give no food, only herbal teas, until the attack has passed. Thyme tea taken alone is excellent for relieving mild asthma.

Because asthma is a serious condition, it is worth visiting a medical herbalist for support and advice, as well as for other effective herbs.

Bach flower remedies Aspen, mimulus or rock rose may help, with others appropriate for underlying emotional problems. Try Rescue Remedy.

Kinesiology Asthma may be related to allergy and anxiety and so respond to the same remedies. In addition, gently rub along the breast bone and lightly touch the anterior fontanelle with two fingertips.

Movement and dance Gentle creative movement can offer general help.

Bites and Stings

Aromatherapy For insect bites and stings in a child over two and a half, apply immediately 1 drop neat essential oil of lavender. If there are several bites or the child is under two and a half, dilute 1 drop lavender oil in a quarter pint of water, stir well and dab on a little. If child is very distressed, pop her into a bath with 1–2 drops lavender (according to age) diluted in 10–20ml of milk. On nettle or garden plant stings, use a cold compress. To 300ml cold water add 2–3 drops lavender. Soak a cloth and apply. Pat dry and apply 1 drop lavender with a clean fingertip.

HOMOEOPATHY FOR BITES AND STINGS

Details of Condition	Remedy
Swelling, shiny, red, swollen lump from a bite that burns or stings. This could either be from a wasp or bee sting or a food allergy	Apis
For animal bites or dirty puncture wounds where the wounded part feels cold. May get twitching of the muscle around the wound	Ledum
The pain is biting, burning, itching and stinging. Hives from an insect bite or stinging nettles. Red, raised blotches with a constant urge to rub	Urtica urens

Bronchitis
• Homoeopathy

Aromatherapy To relieve severe breathing difficulties, try all the methods below for a day, using massage, diffusion and a bath with essential oils. Only use essential oils aggressively like this for up to a week.

Diffuse 2–4 drops of lavender, eucalyptus or tea tree in baby's room for 10 minutes before bed. Massage chest and back sparingly with the following: for one year and over, 2 drops lavender, 1 drop sandalwood to

Bronchitis
(cont.)

30ml almond oil; for under one year, 1–2 drops lavender or 1 drop lavender and 1 drop sandalwood to 30ml almond oil. Diffuse eucalyptus during feeds. Put 1 drop tea tree or lavender on cotton wool ball in her room near radiator or on bed cover (away from contact with the skin). Add 1 drop of tea tree, lavender or sandalwood to a bath. Spray essential oils around the house during virus infections. For children over two and a half, use 1 drop tea tree or eucalyptus to sniff on a tissue occasionally, under supervision. Essential oils sting if too near the eyes.

Movement and dance Once the infection has cleared, creative movement therapy will improve the child's general condition.

Bumps and Bruises
- Colour therapy
- Osteopathy
- Cranio-sacral therapy

Aromatherapy Use a cold compress with 2–3 drops of any of the following essential oils to 300ml water: geranium, cypress or lavender. Agitate water to mix the drops. Lay a compress cloth on bruised area. Repeat as necessary. When the bruise is at the yellow and green stage, massage 10ml carrier oil with 1 drop essential oil of lavender or chamomile gently around bruised area to drain trapped blood. Do not massage active swelling, which must be treated with essential-oil cold compresses only.

Herbalism Apply a cold compress immediately for half an hour to contain any bruising. using neat witch hazel, half a teaspoon of calendula or St John's wort to 275ml water. Infuse daisy, yarrow, hyssop or calendula.

Bach flower remedies Internally, 2 drops Rescue Remedy stirred into a glass of water for the initial shock. Rescue Remedy cream can also be rubbed in. Arnica will deal instantly with bruises.

Kinesiology The ESR technique can soothe any bruised emotions.

Burns and Scalds

Seek medical advice immediately if a burn measures more than 7cm (3in) across, or is very deep, as this could be associated with a severe loss of fluid. Also seek medical attention if the burn becomes more painful or infected.

Aromatherapy Lavender is legendary for taking the sting out of burns and healing quickly without blistering. It also calms distress.

For very minor burns in children over 1 year: if burn is accessible, run under cold water for at least 10 minutes. Apply 1 drop of neat essential oil of lavender. Repeat as needed. Otherwise lay cold compress on area before applying lavender. Cover loosely if necessary. As further treatment of small burns: mix 1 drop lavender into 10ml aloe vera gel and apply. For babies under 1 year: add 2 drops lavender to bowl of very cold water; use as compress. Repeat several times.

Herbalism Immerse the area in cold water for 10 minutes, or until pain subsides. Raise to slow blood flow to the area and ease pain. Do not burst blisters. Apply comfrey ointment, fresh aloe vera juice, St John's wort oil or distilled witch hazel. Infusions of elderflower, plantain, calendula or comfrey can be used as a compress. Repeat frequently. Cover

Burns and Scalds
(cont.)

the area loosely with a clean dry dressing. If it sticks, soak it off with a warm decoction of echinacea or golden seal.

Kinesiology As for bumps and bruises.

HOMOEOPATHY FOR BURNS AND SCALDS	
Purpose	**Remedy**
Prevents blistering and heals burns. You can also use a tincture of the remedy diluted in water to dab on to the burn	Cantharis
Useful if there is ulceration following a burn	Causticum

Catarrh
• Homoeopathy
• Osteopathy
• Cranio-sacral therapy

Naturopathy Exclude milk products, sugar, and refined starchy foods. For persistent catarrh a detox programme may help.

BIOCHEMIC TISSUE SALTS FOR CATARRH	
Remedy	**How to Use**
Natrum mur	3 cellules every two or three hours for watery pale mucus
Kali mur	3 cellules every three hours for thick tenacious mucus
Kali sulph	3 cellules every two or three hours for yellow slimy catarrh

Herbalism Astringent herbs such as plantain, elderflower or yarrow will heal mucous membranes. Herbs high in volatile oils loosen mucus. These include thyme, peppermint, chamomile, cinnamon and ginger. Give one or two from each group, with echinacea, as a hot infusion, a cupful 3–6 times daily, depending on the severity of the problem. For sluggish bowels, cleanse for a week or two with linseed, licorice or dandelion root tea. Garlic perles or raw garlic, daily in honey or salad dressing, clears putrefaction in the bowel, plus catarrh and sinus congestion.

Kinesiology Treat if due to allergy to pasteurized cow's-milk products.

Movement and dance Creative movement readily loosens catarrh.

Chickenpox
(Varicella)
(See over)

Naturopathy In the earliest stages the child will probably lose appetite. Restrict fluids to water and fruit or vegetable juices, given freely. As appetite returns, use fresh juices and fruit, puréed or grated if necessary. Although unlikely, if chickenpox occurs during breast-feeding you

Chickenpox
(cont.)

Try to prevent the infant from scratching the lesions. Seek professional medical help without delay if your child has a fever of 101° F (38.5° C) or more.

- Osteopathy
- Cranio-sacral therapy

should continue as before and be careful with your own diet. In the catarrhal phase continue to avoid dairy products and keep the diet predominantly to vegetables and fruits, either cooked or raw. A slice or two of wholemeal bread, or rice biscuits or some savoury rice or millet may be served with salads or vegetable soups.

Aromatherapy Lotion for children over two years: to 100ml calamine lotion add essential oils in the form of 5 drops German chamomile oil plus 5 drops lavender. Shake well to mix and again before use. Dab on spots with cotton wool.

Herbalism As with all infection you can boost immunity with garlic perles and echinacea, taken every 2 hours (1 garlic perle and from 10 drops to a quarter teaspoon of echinacea tincture). For fever, give hot teas of catnip, yarrow, limeflower or chamomile (half a cupful every 2 hours). If the child is restless, uncomfortable or particularly unhappy, add extra chamomile, catnip or skullcap.

To clear the skin quickly, bring out the rash, and relieve itching, frequently give tea of burdock, chamomile, elderflower or heartsease. Externally, wash with cool infusions of chamomile, chickweed, lavender or marigold, or with distilled witch hazel. If the spots become infected bathe frequently with marigold infusion or dilute tincture.

Homoeopathy There is a homoeopathic prophylactic against chickenpox. It is inadvisable to use this routinely, however, as it is better for the child's immune system for her to have the illness, and increase her defences by building up antibodies. If none of these remedies work, consult your homoeopath.

HOMOEOPATHY FOR CHICKENPOX

Details of Condition	Remedy
Pustular eruptions. Drowsiness, debility and sweat. Rattly mucus but very little coughed up. Child whines if touched. Thirsty for water. White-coated tongue	Antimonium tartaricum
Clingy, weepy, thirstless and better in the open air. Dry cough at night, loose in the morning. Low fever	Pulsatilla
Dry, tickly cough. Intensely itchy eruptions. Restless. Thirsty for milk. Red-tipped tongue	Rhus toxicodendron
Slow recovery. Itching skin which will be red, weepy and worse in heat. Restless, feverish and sweaty. Drinks a lot but eats little	Sulphur

Colds and Flu

Colds are nature's saftety valves. They allow the young system to discharge mucus built up through an accumulation of toxins. In an attack of flu the increased temperature indicates greater defensive activity. Seek professional help without delay if your child has a fever of 101° F (38.5° C) or more.

- Colour therapy
- Osteopathy
- Cranio-sacral therapy

Naturopathy Encourage a diet of juices, fruit, and salads or vegetables. In the early feverish stage, juices and fruit only are best. In the catarrhal stage, keep baby off dairy foods and limit starch intake. With flu, when the temperature is rising, encourage skin activity by tepid sponging of arms, legs, and body (*see page 13*). Use compresses for older children.

A natural vitamin C complex (bioflavonoid), 500mg once or twice daily, may aid recovery. The chewable type is best for young children.

BIOCHEMIC TISSUE SALTS FOR COLDS AND FLU

Remedy	How to Use
Ferrum phos	3 cellules every one or two hours in early feverish stage
Natrum mur	3 cellules every two or three hours for watery nasal discharge
Natrum sulph	3 cellules every three hours for thick, yellowish mucus

Aromatherapy Follow the aromatherapy treatments given for bronchitis.

Herbalism At the first signs give hot infusions of elderflower, yarrow, peppermint, limeflower or chamomile in any combination (half a cupful every 2 hours). These will help to sweat out a fever, resolve infection and clear congestion. Decoctions of ginger or cinnamon can also help. To soothe a sore throat or cough, add plantain, coltsfoot or mullein.

For painful throat and swollen glands, add cleavers or blue flag. For congestion in the chest give thyme, hyssop, elecampane or mullein. Against infection, give echinacea (10 drops to a quarter teaspoon of tincture every 2 hours).

Kinesiology Ensure lots of rest. Encourage sleep, give plenty of fluids and avoid sugar. Exercises support the child's energies and immunity.

HOMOEOPATHY FOR COLDS

Details of Condition	Remedy
Much sneezing, watery nasal discharge, streaming eyes. Worse in a warm room	Allium cepa
Nose blocked, yellow catarrh, irritable. Worse 4 to 8 pm	Lycopodium
Sour taste in mouth. Post-nasal catarrh	Natrum muriaticum

Colds and Flu *(cont.)*

HOMOEOPATHY FOR FLU

Details of Condition	Remedy
Tearing pains. Irritability. Wants to be alone. Worse with slightest movement. Very thirsty. Dry cough, nausea and faint on rising	Bryonia
Aching in bones. Gastric flu. May vomit green bile. Very thirsty	Eupatorium perfoliata
Headache over eye, eyelids heavy. Drowsy, dizzy, trembling. Painful, aching back. Sore throat which can extend to ears. Wants to be alone	Gelsemium

Colic

Common causes of colic are overfeeding and too hasty feeding. You can prevent these by introducing short pauses in the first few minutes of breast-feeding (see page 85 in Part Two). Colic may also be provoked by particular foods, either in the mother's diet if breast-feeding, or in the infant's if weaned. These may be cow's milk, caffeine, wheat, various fruits and spices, yogurt and gassy foods such as turnips and beans. Goat's milk or soya milk may be preferable to cow's. Anxiety and stress may be contributory factors.

- Osteopathy
- Cranio-Sacral therapy

Naturopathy Simmer 1 dessertspoonful of dill seed in boiling water for 15 minutes. Strain, and serve by bottle as required.

Abdominal discomfort may be relieved by hot fomentations.

Massage Regular massage in the early evening will help. Use the sequence from Chapter Two (*see pages 76–8*), but include more strokes over the abdomen. Massage the belly down towards the groin, one hand following the other repeatedly. Move your hand(s) clockwise over the baby's tummy. Start at the lower right, going up the centre and down on the left. Use one hand on a small area, perhaps placing the other on top, as your baby gets older. If you suspect constipation, this helps eliminate waste as you follow the direction of the colon.

Lightly make small circles with your fingertips over the same area. Use the paddling stroke again. Lift up the baby's legs, bending them at the knee and press them gently towards her abdomen.

Aromatherapy Massage using Roman chamomile oil – excellent for colic.

Herbalism Before feeds, 25ml herbal infusion, a quarter to a half teaspoon of herb to 100ml boiling water: try catnip, lemon balm, fennel, dill, chamomile or marshmallow. Add the same infusions to baths. Take an adult dose if breast-feeding. Before feeds, give a warm bath with infusions. A tense breast-feeding mother may cause the baby spasms in the gut. Give teas or tinctures of relaxing herbs such as skullcap, vervain, chamomile, lemon balm, hops or limeflower, 3–6 times daily.

Bach flower remedies Aspen, mimulus, rock rose or white chestnut may be useful. Try walnut for the baby.

Kinesiology Give gentle, soothing, rocking movements and soft rhythmical sound. Try gently rubbing along the outside and inside of the thighs.

Alexander technique If practised regularly by the mother this can diminish the frequency and intensity of colic.

Colic (cont.)

HOMOEOPATHY TO TREAT COLIC

Details of Condition	Remedy
Often triggered by anger. Child bends over double with pain and draws legs up. Eased by pressure and warmth. Eating and drinking causes a dysenteric-type stool	Colocynthis
Intolerant of pain; condition often accompanies teething. One red cheek, one white. Green mucousy stools. Child cries out when passing stool. Angry and wants to be carried. Capricious	Chamomilla
Child arches back and screams. Rumbly abdomen. Better upright	Dioscorea
Worse after fruit. Smelly, loud wind; better for passing it. Stool smelly and thin	Natrum sulphuricum
This remedy may be needed in breast-fed babies where the mother has consumed too much spicy food or something too stimulating such as tea or coffee. Cramping, griping pains. Better for passing stool but worse for eating. Bad-tempered child. Chilly	Nux vomica
Bloated, tight stomach. Stools olive green. This may happen in very young babies whose mothers have had the drug Syntometrin to remove the placenta. Secale will antidote the ill effects on the baby	Secale

Constipation

It is important not to get anxious about your child's stools. Each of us has a different rhythm and left to themselves the bowels move whenever they need to.

• Homoeopathy
• Kinesiology
• Osteopathy
• Cranio-sacral therapy

Naturopathy Establish regular toilet times. Apply hot fomentations to the abdomen for 10 or 15 minutes beforehand. Give soluble fibre such as grated apples or carrot, and ripe bananas on an empty stomach.

Grind one teaspoonful of flax seed and serve on fruit or cereal or swallow with water. For breast- or bottle-feeding babies, give 1 teaspoonful of honey in warm water on an empty stomach twice daily.

Massage Bowel movements can be helped by clockwise massage of the baby's tummy, and massage around the anus stimulates rectal muscles.

If baby is small, use one hand; otherwise use two, one following the other in a smooth rhythm. Use a small quantity of warm oil and firm pressure. Make small circular movements with the fingertips to assist the natural movement of waste matter. Then, with flat hands stroke down from under the ribcage towards the groin, one hand again following the other. Try placing the heel of your hand under the anus. Lightly press in a small circular motion for a couple of minutes.

Aromatherapy Constipation is common in children being bottle fed or toilet trained. Give frequent drinks of water or dilute fruit juice. Massage the lower abdomen and lower back, using 1 drop essential oil of chamomile and 1 drop mandarin in 20–30ml almond oil. Use a little

Constipation (cont.)

of the oil twice a day for 3–4 days. A warm bath with 1–2 drops essential oil of lavender diluted in milk can be very comforting.

Movement and dance Creative movement can work wonders.

Herbalism Treatment will depend on the cause, which could be diet, allergy, tension, upset of bacterial population of gut, lack of exercise, vitamin and mineral imbalance or insufficient fluids.

HERBAL TREATMENT FOR CONSTIPATION

Purpose	Herbal remedy
To balance bacterial population of the gut	Garlic, live yogurt, olive oil or thyme tea
To bulk out the stool	Psyllium seeds, flax seeds: take half to 1 teaspoonful in a cup of warm water. Allow to swell into a gel and give before bed
To stimulate bowels and encourage liver function	Dandelion root, yellow dock root or burdock root, 2–3 times daily
To soothe an irritated gut and lubricate the stool	Marshmallow, slippery elm or comfrey leaf
For anxious children, to relax bowel muscles	Chamomile, lemon balm, hops, catnip, fennel or dill

Cough
• Homoeopathy
• Osteopathy
• Cranio-sacral therapy

Naturopathy Avoid mucus-forming foods like milk and cheese; limit animal protein. Give half teaspoonful honey with juice of half a lemon in warm water. Apply hot fomentation to chest and upper back. Rub Olbas oil on chest and throat. Give 3 cellules Kali mur 2–3 hourly.

Herbalism
DRY COUGH WITH FEVER Give elecampane, thyme, hyssop and garlic; and for the fever, yarrow, elderflower, limeflower, chamomile or catnip. Expectorant herbs include thyme, coltsfoot and mullein.

CATARRHAL COUGH Stimulating expectorant herbs to shift phlegm: cinnamon, ginger, hyssop, thyme, horehound or elecampane.

DRY IRRITATING COUGH Soothe, and loosen phlegm, with coltsfoot, lungwort, mullein, comfrey leaf, marshmallow, or cowslip flowers.

Bach flower remedies Use Dr Bach's rock rose or Rescue Remedy if a child becomes distressed during coughing bouts.

Cough (cont.)

Kinesiology A cough with abundant mucus may be linked to an allergy. Maintain a warm humid atmosphere. Rub along the length of the breast bone and lightly hold with the tips of two fingers the anterior fontanelle.

Movement and dance Creative movement loosens catarrh in a cough.

Cradle Cap

This scurf condition, also known as milk cap, occurs on the scalp of babies who have an allergic disposition or are constitutionally inclined to lymphatic congestion and catarrh.

Naturopathy If breast-feeding, avoid sugar, refined carbohydrates and dairy foods. Seek professional advice for constitutional remedies.

Aromatherapy Massage the following into the scalp for 1–2 days: under one year, for essential oil use 1 drop rose and 1 drop chamomile to 30ml almond oil; over one year, use 1 drop rose and 1 drop chamomile to 20ml almond oil. Shampoo: add 1–2 drops essential oil of tea tree to 30–50ml baby shampoo. Shake well. Apply only a small amount. Avoid the eyes and rinse well. Use for 1–2 weeks or until scalp clears.

Herbalism Rub the scalp regularly with olive oil before bed. Wash off the loosened crusts the following morning with natural-based shampoo and rinse with cider vinegar added to the water. Afterwards, bathe with a lotion of heartsease, meadowsweet or burdock infusion. (Never pick off crusts that have not loosened, as this may cause bleeding and infection.)

HOMOEOPATHY TO TREAT CRADLE CAP

Details of Condition	Remedy
Sweaty baby with sour-smelling thick crusts on the head	Calcerea carbonica
Thin, whiny baby. Flatulence between 4 and 8 pm	Lycopodium
Dry, itchy cradle cap. Hot baby. Thirsty and prefers drinking to eating. Loves sweet-tasting foods	Sulphur

Crying
• Homoeopathy
• Alexander technique
• Osteopathy
• Cranio-sacral therapy

Herbalism To encourage restful sleep, add strong infusions to a bath; for example, chamomile, catnip, cowslip, hops, lavender, lemon balm or limeflower. Before bed, massage the feet, abdomen or head with any of the above (diluted), or use oils in a vaporizer in the room. Give dilute teas of any of these on a spoon or in a bottle.

Bach flower remedies Try aspen, mimulus, rock rose, holly, sweet chestnut or Rescue Remedy.

Bates method Cradle the baby and rock gently. An inconsolable state can cause fixation in seeing, so when crying stops, renew movement by play. Show one of the following colours: red, yellow, white, blue or green.

Crying (cont.)

Kinesiology All crying needs loving observation in order to understand the message. Expert help may be needed, in case of a serious problem (*see page 85*). Rhythmical movement and soft music may offer relief.

Movement and dance Creative movement helps release frustration.

Cuts and Grazes

You may need to close the cut with surgical tape. If it is deep or there is risk of tetanus, seek medical advice.

Aromatherapy Essential oils of tea tree and lavender are both antiseptic, antibiotic and antifungal. Wash and clean wound with 2–3 drops lavender or tea tree diluted in 300ml water. Cover cut with gauze. Clean with lavender as necessary. Use healing gel if needed.

Healing cream gel: to a 50g pot of aloe vera gel add 6 drops lavender and 6 drops tea tree oil. Add 10 per cent calendula oil. Mix well.

Herbalism Clean the area well with herbal antiseptic to prevent infection and speed healing. Use 4–5 drops of tincture of myrrh, golden seal, St John's wort or calendula in warm water to wash the area. Cover with a dressing of cream with St John's wort, comfrey, or calendula.

Bach flower remedies Give Rescue Remedy or Star of Bethlehem for the shock of the initial accident.

Homoeopathy Use hypercal tincture, made from hypericum and calendula. Dilute 10 drops in a mug of warm water. Apply with cotton wool.

Colour therapy Your therapist will apply turquoise solarized cream.

Kinesiology Ease pain and support circulation with exercises.

Diarrhoea

It is important to determine the cause of the diarrhoea before treating. Seek professional medical help without delay if the condition persists for more than 48 hours. Meanwhile give as much fluid as possible.

- Osteopathy
- Cranio-sacral therapy

Naturopathy Give plenty of fluids, vegetable broths, grated raw apples and steamed vegetables, such as carrots or cauliflower. Rice water (from boiled rice) helps to stabilize minerals and prevent dehydration.

As emergency recipe tso control prolonged diarrhoea: 1 cupful of boiled milk sprinkled with 1 teaspoonful of grated nutmeg. For very small children: stir-fry 3–10g of hazelnut kernels to blacken surface, crush to powder, cover with water and simmer for 15–20 minutes. Give the liquid 3 times daily. After the acute phase reintroduce rice, steamed vegetables (puréed if necessary) and live goat's or sheep's yogurt.

BIOCHEMIC TISSUE SALTS FOR DIARRHOEA

Remedy	How to Use
Natrum mur	3 cellules every half hour for watery stools causing soreness
Calc phos	3 cellules half hourly for teething children with hot, watery or greenish stools and undigested food

Diarrhoea
(cont.)

Aromatherapy Give the child a warm bath with 1 drop chamomile, sandalwood or lavender (diluted in milk). Gentle massage also helps ease cramping pain. For babies under one year: use 2 drops chamomile to 30ml carrier oil; for children over one year: use one of the formulae below according to cause. Use sparingly once or twice a day.

Food or viral bacterial infections: for essential oils use 1 drop chamomile and 1 drop lavender, to 20ml carrier oil. Diffuse 1 drop peppermint in baby's room. This essential oil should never be used in a child's bath or on her skin and with caution in adults as it stings.

Emotional cause: use 1 drop essential oil of chamomile and 1 drop essential oil of mandarin or neroli to 20ml carrier oil, to massage the lower abdomen in a gentle clockwise motion.

Herbalism Chamomile, thyme, ginger or fennel can be given in tea. They are mildly antiseptic and help to relax the bowel and relieve griping. If diarrhoea is severe or prolonged, use astringent herbs such as agrimony, meadowsweet, tormentil or shepherd's purse, combined with carminative herbs such as cinnamon, fennel, ginger and peppermint, in teas or tinctures 3–6 times daily depending on whether chronic or acute.

Give garlic every 2 hours in acute infections. In addition slippery elm powder can be made into a soothing gruel by adding water.

Homoeopathy If the child is on solids, keep her on a diet of porridge made with water, plain boiled rice, and grated apple mixed with a little live yogurt. Also rice cakes. Give water to drink.

HOMOEOPATHY TO TREAT DIARRHOEA

Details of Condition	Remedy
Diarrhoea comes on at midnight with fear, anxiety about dying, and restlessness and weakness. Triggered by bad meat or watery fruits. Child may want sips of water; desires company	Arsenicum album
Green diarrhoea that accompanies teething. Child irritable. One red cheek, one pale. Child consoled by being carried	Chamomilla
Sudden onset in oversensitive child. Fear of dark. Wants company, cold drinks, ice cream. Often vomiting	Phosphorous

Kinesiology If allergies are suspected, avoid trigger foods. For emotional causes use ESR technique. Stroke the fingers together over the left cheekbone and gently rub the outside and insides of the thighs.

Ear Infections

Severe earache should be referred to a doctor. Consult a naturopath for constitutional and long-term management, especially attention to lymphatic drainage. Seek professional medical help without delay if your child has a fever of 101° F (38.5° C) or more.

- Homoeopathy
- Osteopathy
- Cranio-sacral therapy

Naturopathy Juice fast and cleansing diet. Avoid cow's milk, sugar, refined carbohydrates. Apply warm grated carrot poultice to relieve pain and encourage discharge. Give 3 cellules of Kali sulph every 3–4 hours, for catarrhal discharges from ear with pain beneath.

FOR EARACHE Short juice fast on carrot, beet and cucumber juice or carrot, celery and parsley juice. Follow with vegetable broths or soups and steamed vegetables. Raw fruit and salads for older children. Chewing carrots or apples will stimulate lymph glands and relieve congestion in the Eustachian tube connecting the ear and throat.

Place a little warm olive oil in the ear and plug with cotton wool overnight. Make an infusion of peppermint tea and allow the steam to enter the ear. Also make a poultice of raw grated carrot in a gauze chamber, steep in hot water and apply behind and below the ear, especially if there are swollen glands. Give 3 cellules Ferrum phos every 1–2 hours for earache with fever, pain, congestion, and throbbing.

Aromatherapy

FOR EARACHE AND MIDDLE EAR INFECTION Make a compress, adding 2–3 drops essential oil of Roman chamomile to 300ml hot water. Mix to disperse oils. Lay cloth on top. Squeeze out; hold against ear. To massage round ear and neck, use as essential oils 1 drop Roman chamomile and 1 drop lavender, to 20–30ml almond oil, according to age.

Herbalism

FOR ACUTE MIDDLE EAR INFECTION If there is no pus in the ear and the drum has not perforated, apply a few drops of warmed olive oil, plugged with cotton wool. Give teas or tinctures to relax and soothe, combined with antiseptic herbs such as chamomile, echinacea and hyssop, with relaxant herbs (chamomile or skullcap), and remedies for catarrhal congestion, such as elderflower, ground ivy or yarrow.

FOR RECURRENT MIDDLE EAR INFECTION AND GLUE EAR It is important to treat the underlying problem, such as chronic catarrh, low resistance to infections, poor diet, passive smoking, stress or allergy.

Herbs for the immune system: chamomile, echinacea, hyssop or peppermint; herbs to clear catarrh: chamomile, hyssop, elderflower, yarrow or plantain; herbs to decongest tonsils and lymph glands: cleavers or marigold. Give garlic daily in food, perles or raw in salad.

Kinesiology Help with exercises. Hold a palm over the baby's ear and the thumb and two fingers of the other hand over the ESR points.

Glue ear affects fewer children who are breast-fed. There may also be a link with food allergies, cow's-milk products and sugar.

Eczema

Eczema may be caused by allergy, stress, bottle milk formula, or external irritants such as washing powder, wool or chlorinated water.

- Aromatherapy
- Homoeopathy
- Cranio-sacral therapy

Naturopathy Avoid food allergens: exclude cow's milk, cheese, sugar, and citrus fruits. Short juice fasts or cleansing diet, followed by steamed vegetables and vegetable soups. Juices of carrot, beet and cucumber, or cucumber, endive and pineapple. Increase essential fatty acids with tahini, sunflower or pumpkin seeds, and blackcurrant seed oil.

Applications: Oatmeal bath – place 500g uncooked oatmeal in a gauze bag, soak in a bath of warm water or mix the oatmeal in the water. Soak the baby in the bath for 10–15 minutes.

Raspberry wash – take 250g fresh raspberries (if in season), add water and simmer to thick liquid. Wash affected area three times daily.

Herbalism Use herbs as warm teas rather than tinctures for skin problems. Externally, use evening primrose oil, aloe vera gel, vitamin E oil, chamomile cream, comfrey cream or calendula cream.

Bath the child with infusions of marigold, chamomile, yarrow, chickweed or burdock.

HERBAL TREATMENT FOR ECZEMA

Purpose	Remedy
To boost immunity	Chamomile, echinacea, nettles, red clover, yarrow
To cool and nourish the blood	Burdock, heartsease, nettles, red clover, fumitory
To treat stress add herbs to support the nervous system	Chamomile, vervain, wild oats, skullcap

Kinesiology Use the ESR technique for emotional disturbance. More complete relief needs skilled professional help.

Movement and dance Creative movement helps dissipate any anxiety.

Eye Infections

- Homoeopathy
- Osteopathy
- Cranio-sacral therapy

Herbalism

STYES Apply warm compress for a few minutes every 2–3 hours to help bring stye to a head; use decoction or infusion of burdock, chamomile, elderflower, eyebright, marigold or marshmallow; or 5 drops of tincture in half a cup of distilled water, with rosewater or witch hazel. Give teas three times daily, to detoxify the system and increase resistance, using echinacea, burdock, eyebright, garlic or red clover.

CONJUNCTIVITIS Bathe the eyes three times daily with a decoction of elderflower, eyebright, marigold, chamomile or plantain. Tea bags of these (or Indian tea) can be soaked in boiling water and used, lukewarm,

Eye Infections (cont.)

for 5–10 minutes, with a different bag for each eye so as not to spread the infection. You can add rose water to any of these decoctions. Always ensure the eye bath is sterilized or, if using cotton wool, apply a different piece to each eye and wipe inwards towards the nose.

Give herbs to enhance immunity; for example, chamomile, marigold, thyme, echinacea, hyssop and eyebright, singly or combined.

If your child suffers frequently from conjunctivitis, consult a medical herbalist about diet, allergies, rundown state of health, stress.

Homoeopathy Bathe the eyes with cooled boiled water to which 5 drops of hypercal tincture have been added. In persistent cases use one of the following remedies.

HOMOEOPATHY FOR EYE INFECTIONS

Details of Condition	Remedy
Pus, sometimes smell, discharge from the eye. Accompanies a cold. Eyelids glued together. Child generally cold, stubborn, sluggish. Sour-smelling sweat on head	Calcarea carbonica
Burning, watery discharge. Eyes water in the light. Eyelids red and swollen. Better for cold	Euphrasia
Purulent, smelly, thick, yellow discharge. Worse at night and in the cold, better for fresh air. Child whiny, clingy. Thirstless	Pulsatilla

Bates method Eye infections may result from difficulties in the immune system or from fatigue, and may be connected to allergies. You can treat as for allergy, as well as using some of the procedures listed in Part Two (*see pages 83–4, 97–8, 109, 119, 130 and 137*) to encourage relaxation and easy seeing. Be aware of any irritation caused by too-bright light.

Kinesiology Eye infections (including conjunctivitis) may indicate deep-seated problems as well as local irritation, which may be caused by fluorescent lights. Also, the tear ducts may be blocked.

Relieve by stroking downwards on either side of the nose from its root. Also softly run the pads of the fingers around the orbits of the eyes, out over the eyebrows and in under the eyes.

Lightly touch with two fingertips a point in front of the ears. You can identify this as being immediately above the bone. Touch another point just outside the outer tip of the eyebrows, either alone or in conjunction with the ESR points. Avoid harsh light. You may find it soothing to look at a blue colour.

Hyperactivity

Adopt a diet free of allergens and especially avoid sugar, colas, and foods with chemical and colouring additives.

- Homoeopathy
- Alexander technique
- Osteopathy
- Cranio-sacral therapy

Rash

(Including Nappy)
Find the cause: it may be a certain soap or soap powder. Nappy rash can be provoked by a chemical in disposable nappies, from not washing the child regularly, or from not changing the nappy often enough.

Naturopathy Stabilize blood sugar levels with regular, well-balanced meals, and savoury snacks (such as sunflower seeds, nuts, rice biscuits with savoury spread) between the main meals to prevent energy dips. Give the Biochemic Tissue Salts: Kali phos and Mag phos – 3 cellules four times daily.

Herbalism The causes need to be ascertained by a medical herbalist: allergy, nutritional deficiency, emotional causes, passive smoking, candida, or accumulation of heavy metals, for example. Red clover, kelp and nettles help cleanse the latter. Combine with tonic herbs to support the nerves and adrenal glands, such as skullcap, vervain, wild oats, borage and licorice. To aid sleep you may need to give relaxing herbs such as chamomile, catnip, hops or limeflower.

Bach flower remedies Vervain, impatiens, holly, aspen or walnut.

Movement and dance Creative playtime is one of the best natural therapies through which to release a phenomenal energy.

Naturopathy Breast-feeding mothers should reduce animal proteins and exclude sweet foods and citrus fruits from their own diet or the child's after weaning. Persistent cases may be helped by a cleansing diet of steamed rice or millet, and vegetables which can be puréed.

Aromatherapy Sore skin needs the air. For nappy rash, allow plenty of free playtime without nappies. Add 1–2 drops chamomile or lavender diluted in milk to baby's bath water. If rash is caused by thrush, as an essential oil substitute 1 drop tea tree instead of lavender or chamomile.

Cream lotion: to 50g pot unperfumed, lanolin-free cream, add 3 drops German chamomile and 3 drops lavender. For thrush, substitute 3 drops tea tree for the lavender. Calendula oil 10 per cent will help heal skin. (Calendula oil here is a 'base' or carrier oil – not an essential oil.)

During nappy changes jojoba oil is excellent as it leaves a fine waxy coating which moisturizes and soothes. Apply a little of the following: to 30ml jojoba carrier oil add 1 drop rose and 1 drop lavender or 1 drop lavender and 1 drop Roman chamomile. If skin is very sore, use 10 per cent calendula carrier oil in the blend. Where there is no rash, use the standard baby massage formula, 50ml carrier with 2 drops essential oil.

Herbalism Ascertain causes: stress, allergies, wounds, sunburn, plants, washing powder, infection, deficient diet, animal dander, antibiotics.

To relieve inflammation, bathe with an infusion of wild pansy, yellow dock, burdock or chickweed, or add strong infusion to bath water and soak for half an hour. To clear toxins, give herbs such as cleavers, red clover, heartsease, fumitory, burdock, marigold, nettles or dandelion

Rash (cont.)

leaves. Also add herbs to enhance the immune system: echinacea or wild indigo. To support the adrenal glands, add borage or licorice.

To reduce stress, add chamomile, limeflower, vervain or skullcap. For nappy rash, at each change wash with herbal infusions of lavender, marigold, or chamomile. Alternatively, use dilute witch hazel or neat rose water. Dry thoroughly and apply a cream of comfrey, chamomile, marigold or chickweed. If you suspect thrush, use marigold, golden seal or chamomile cream. Egg white, repeatedly applied and allowed to dry, builds up a protective layer of albumen.

Bach flower remedies Give aspen, mimulus, crab apple or agrimony.

Homoeopathy Where there is great redness, try a few doses of Sulphur. If this does not help, consult your homoeopath. Apply calendula or Rescue cream and leave nappy off as often as possible.

Colour therapy Your therapist will treat with yellow solarized cream.

Kinesiology Avoid any suspected irritants. Seek professional help, and assist cleansing with exercises.

Sleepless-ness

This has many causes: fear, worry, threat, illness, diet or allergy. Check to see if sibling rivalry is a factor.

- Homoeopathy
- Colour therapy
- Osteopathy
- Cranio-sacral therapy

Naturopathy Avoid stimulation at bedtime. Give carbohydrate-based suppers: pastas and grains, bananas, or warm drinks with honey. Before bed, sponge or spray the legs and feet with cool water and dry.

Massage Massage as for colic (*see pages 76–7*). Do not give sedative drugs. Take baby into bed with you to help her relax.

Aromatherapy Massage with dilute oils of chamomile, lavender, neroli or rose just before sleep.

Herbalism Causes must be known before treatment; hyperactivity, anxiety, allergy, nutritional deficiencies, candida, overtiredness, lack of fresh air and exercise, fever, illness, irritation of skin or rash are possibilities.

Add strong infusions of catnip, chamomile, limeflower, hops, passionflower or lemon balm to bath. Give a cup of warm tea before bed, using chamomile, catnip, cowslip flowers, lemon balm or limeflower. If emotional problems or stress are contributing, give herbs 3 times daily during the day to support the nervous system; for example, skullcap, lemon balm, St John's wort, vervain and wild oats.

Bach flower remedies Give these during the day, before bed, and again if the child wakes. Use aspen, mimulus, walnut or white chestnut.

Colour therapy Your therapist will prescribe.pink in clothes or a cover.

Bates method Relaxing games, story telling, palming and rocking.

Kinesiology Remove obvious stresses. Help with exercises.

Movement and dance Regular creative movement can promote sleep.

Sunburn

Keep young children out of the sun and protect with hats and Factor 20 sun cream. Give plenty of fluids. Seek urgent medical advice if burning is severe or the child has a bad headache and double vision.

- Colour therapy
- Alexander technique
- Cranio-sacral therapy

Aromatherapy Make a cold compress, adding 1–2 drops essential oil of lavender to 300ml water, and lay on the inflamed area. Alternatively, to 300ml cool water add 2–3 drops lavender, and spray frequently.

You can also immerse the child in a coolish bath to which has been added 1–2 drops lavender oil depending on age. Take a small towel, squeeze it out in the bath water, and lay it across the child's shoulders to help cool her. Gently pat the child dry, keep her quiet, and give her plenty of clear fluids to drink.

Repeat the bath in 2 hours if necessary.

Herbalism Treat the skin liberally with cucumber juice to soothe. A tepid infusion of lavender, nettle, elderflower or chamomile, in water or milk, can be soothing and healing. Aloe vera juice, potato juice, black tea, distilled witch hazel, natural yogurt, or 1 teaspoonful of cider vinegar in 30ml of water or a mixture of olive oil and glycerine, can also be used for cooling the skin.

Homoeopathy Sol 30 should be given prophylactically.

Kinesiology Support recovery with exercises.

Teething

The rate of teething differs from one baby to another. Some will be born with a tooth, others may still be toothless at one year old. Your baby may have no sign other than a slightly red gum and a pink spot on the cheeks.

- Cranio-sacral therapy

Massage Try simple massage with no creams or oils. Circle a thumb or fingertip gently at the front, behind, and along the gum, for one minute a day. This helps circulation and may ease the tooth's progress.

Herbalism Chewing on marshmallow root or licorice stick is soothing and antiflammatory. Rub gums with glycerine or honey. Give frequent infusions of chamomile, limeflower, yarrow, fennel or catnip.

Kinesiology Gently rub the tissue around the jaw, and help with exercises.

HOMOEOPATHY FOR TEETHING

Details of Condition	Remedy
Hot, red, swollen cheeks, restless sleep. May be feverish	Belladonna
Sour sweat on head. Cold baby with slow, painful teething	Calcarea carbonica
Irritable, restless child who likes to be carried. One red cheek and one pale. Green stools	Chamomilla
Whiny and clingy. Feels better out of doors. Thirstless	Pulsatilla

Tonsillitis

Seek professional medical help without delay if your child has a fever of 101° F (38.5° C) or more.

- Osteopathy
- Cranio-sacral therapy

Naturopathy Short juice fast. Exclude mucus-forming foods – milk products, sugar, refined carbohydrates. Vegetable soups and puréed vegetables. Cold throat and abdominal compress for children over 18 months. Treat with Biochemic Tissue Salts: Ferrum phos – 3 cellules every 1–2 hours for early feverish flushed phase; Kali mur – 3 cellules every 3–4 hours for advanced stage with swollen glands and pain on swallowing.

Herbalism At least one herb per category, in tea every 2 hours. To help immunity, give echinacea, garlic or thyme. Cleavers and marigold support lymphatic tissue in cleansing. To reduce fever you should give chamomile, catnip, elderflower, limeflower or yarrow. To tone the mucous membranes and clear catarrh and inflammation, use plantain, elderflower, ground ivy or raspberry leaves; and to soothe and relieve painful tonsils, dose with coltsfoot, mullein, or marshmallow. Gargles or sprays can be made from infusions of half a teaspoonful of tincture, and warm water, of ground ivy, sage, thyme, or chamomile.

Homoeopathy Belladonna, for: red cheeks; heat with icy feet; glazed eyes; dilated pupils, maybe hallucinations; sore tonsils; thirstlessness.

Kinesiology Try exercises.

Travel Sickness

- Homoeopathy
- Osteopathy
- Cranio-sacral therapy

Naturopathy Beforehand, avoid feeding any dairy, fatty, or starchy foods. Give light meals of fruit or vegetable soups (*see Part One, page 12*).

Aromatherapy To 30ml almond oil add 1 drop essential oil of mandarin. Mix; massage over upper abdomen before journey. Sprinkle 1–2 drops peppermint oil on tissues or damp cotton wool. Put one on dashboard shelf, another in the back out of child's reach. For a child over two and a half, sprinkle 1 drop ginger on tissue to inhale. Do not use these essential oils on children's skin as they may irritate. For babies, massage feet with 1–3 drops essential oil of chamomile in 30ml almond oil.

Herbalism Offer fresh ginger, crystallized ginger, ginger beer or decoction, or a few drops of tincture. Peppermint and meadowsweet teas also help. For nerves, use catnip, chamomile, passionflower or skullcap.

Kinesiology Help baby with exercises.

Vomiting

If prolonged or violent, or your child's temperature is 101° F (38.5° C) or more, get swift medical help.

Naturopathy Vomiting can accompany catarrhal disorders (tonsillitis, whooping cough) or digestive disturbances. A short juice fast, or a bland diet of foods such as grated or puréed apple or puréed vegetables and vegetable soups.

Take care to prevent inhalation of vomit.

Kinesiology Rehydrate with cool boiled water, support with exercises.

Useful Addresses

COMPLEMENTARY THERAPIES

General Organizations

British Complementary Medical Association (BCMA)
39 Prestbury Road
Pittville
Cheltenham GL52 2PT
Tel: 01242 226770

Institute for Complementary Medicine / British Register of Complementary Practitioners
Tavern Quay
Plough Way
Surrey Quays
London SE16 1QZ
Tel: 0171 237 5165

Complementary Medicine Association
Unit 5, 9 Packard Avenue
PO Box 727
Castle Hill
NSW 2154
Tel: 02 894 5581
Fax: 02 899 5513

Alexander Technique

Alexander Technique Network
PO Box 53
Kendal
Cumbria
LA9 4UP

The Society of Teachers of the Alexander Technique
20 London House
266 Fulham Road
London SW10 9EL
Tel: 0171 351 0828

The Australian Society of Teachers of the Alexander Technique
PO Box 716
Darlinghurst
NSW 2010

SATA
16 Princess Street
Kew
Victoria 3101
Tel: 03 853 1356
(Toll Free: 008 339 571)
Fax: 03 859 5929

Aromatherapy

The International Federation of Aromatherapists
Stamford House
2/4 Chiswick High Road
London W4 1TH
Tel: 0181 742 2605

Allison England Aromatherapy
The Trees
97 Main Street
Little Downham
Ely, Cambridgeshire
CB6 2SX
Tel/Fax: 01353 699236
(Supplier of pure and blended essential oils, with special mother and baby range)

Aromatherapy Clinic of Sydney
1 O'Connell Street
Sydney
NSW 2000
Tel: 02 241 4030
Fax: 02 241 4270

Bates Method

The Bates Association of Great Britain
PO Box 25
Shoreham by Sea
W. Sussex BN43 6ZF

Bates/Kinesiology
Anthony Attenborough
128 Merton Road
London SW18 5SP
Tel/Fax: 0181 874 7337

Natural Vision Improvement
Janet Goodrich
Crystal Waters Permaculture Village
MS–16, Maleny
Queensland 4552
Tel: 74 944657
Fax: 74 944673

Colour Therapy

International Association for Colour Therapy
The Chairwoman
137 Hendon Lane
London N3 3PR
Tel: 0181 349 3299

Colour and Reflexology

Pauline Wills
9 Wyndale Avenue
Kingsbury
London NW9 9PT
Tel: 0181 204 7672

Aura-Soma Australia
Harry and Margaret Simon
10 Cygnet Place
Illawong
NSW 2234
Tel: 02 541 1066
Fax: 02 543 0240

Cranio–Sacral Therapy

The Cranio-Sacral Therapy Association
The Secretary
Stillpoint
Whiteway, Stroud
Gloucestershire
GL6 7EP
Tel: 01285 821648

The College of Cranio-Sacral Therapy
9 St George's Mews
Primrose Hill
London NW1 8XE
Tel: 0171 483 0120

Herbalism

General Council and Register of Consultant Herbalists
18 Sussex Square
Brighton
E. Sussex BM2 5AA

National Institute of Medical Herbalists
56 Longbrook Street
Exeter EX4 6AH
Tel: 01392 426022

The Herb Society of South Australia
PO Box 140
Parkside
South Australia 5063
Tel/Fax: 08 345 3808

National Herbalists Association of Australia
PO Box 65
249 Kingsgrove Road

Kingsgrove
NSW 2208
Tel: 02 502 2938
Fax: 02 554 3459

Homoeopathy

British Homoeopathic Association
27a Devonshire Street
London W1N 1RJ
Tel: 0171 935 2163

Society of Homoeopaths
2 Artizan Road
Northampton NN1 4HU
Tel: 01604 21400

Australian Federation of Homoeopaths
7/29 Bertram Street
Chatswood
NSW 2067
Tel: 02 415 3928

Kinesiology

Association of Systematic Kinesiology
39 Browns Road
Surbiton
Surrey KT5 8ST
Tel: 0181 399 3215
Fax: 0181 399 1010

The Kinesiology Federation
The TFH Centre
30 Sudley Road
Bognor Regis
W. Sussex PO21 1ER
Tel: 0243 841689

Australian Kinesiology Association
PO Box 190
East Kew
Victoria 3102
Tel: 03 859 2254

Educational Kinesiology Foundation
c/o Tania McGregor
Dynamic Living Centre
218 Glen Osmond Road
Fullarton
South Australia 5063
Tel: 08 379 6988
Fax: 08 379 0942

Massage

British Massage Therapy Council (BMTC)
Greenbank House
65a Adelphi Street
Preston
Lancashire PR1 7BH
Tel: 01772 881063

London College of Massage
5 Newman Passage
London W1P 3PN
Tel: 0171 323 3574
(For courses in holistic massage)

Association of Remedial Masseurs
Suite 1
120 Blaxland Road
Ryde
NSW 2112
Tel: 02 807 4769

Movement and Dance

The Medau Society
8b Robson House
East Street
Epsom
Surrey KT17 1HH
Tel: 01372 729056

Lucy Jackson
23 Springfield Road
London NW8 0JQ
Tel: 0171 624 3580
(Teacher of Medau Method)

Naturopathy

British Naturopathic Association
Frazer House
6 Netherhall Gardens
London NW3 5RR
Tel: 0171 435 8728

Australian Natural Therapists Association
PO Box 856
Caloundra
Queensland 4551
Tel (Toll Free): 008 817 577

Osteopathy

British and European Osteopathic Association
6 Adelaide Road
Teddington
Middlesex TW11 0AY
Tel: 0181 977 8532

Osteopathic Information Service
PO Box 2074
Reading
Berkshire RG1 4YR
Tel: 01734 512051

Australian Osteopathic Association
PO Box 699
Turramurra
NSW 2074
Tel: 02 449 4799
Fax: 02 449 6587

Sound Therapy

Association of Professional Music Therapists in Great Britain
48 Lancaster Road
London N6 4TA

Olivea Dewhurst-Maddock
47 Kentsford Road
Kents Bank
Grange-over-Sands
Cumbria LA11 7BB
(For courses on Sound Therapy)

Bibliography

Balaskas, Arthur and Walker, Peter, *Baby Gymnastics*. London: Unwin Paperbacks, 1985

Balaskas, Janet and Gordon, Yehudi, *Pregnancy and Birth*. London: Little, Brown and Company, 1992

Barhydt, Elizabeth and Hamilton, *Self-help for Kids*. Groveland, CA: Loving Life, 1992

Bates, William H. m.d., *Better Eyesight Without Glasses*. London: Grafton Books, Collins Publishing Group, 1988

Birth to Five. London: The Health Education Authority, 1994

Bower, Tom, *The Perceptual World of the Child*. Glasgow: Fontana, 1977

Brennan, Richard, *The Alexander Technique Manual*. London: Little, Brown and Company, 1996, and Sydney: Simon and Schuster, 1996

Brennan, Richard, *The Alexander Technique Workbook*. Dorset: Element Books, 1992

Butler, Brian, *Kinesiology for Balanced Health*. Surbiton, Surrey: TASK Books, 1992

Castro, Miranda, *Homeopathy for Mother and Baby*. New York: Macmillan, 1992

Dennison, Gail and Paul Ph.D, *Edu-K for Kids*. Ventura, CA: Edu-Kinesthetics, 1987

Dewhurst-Maddock, Olivea, *The Book of Sound Therapy*. London: Gaia Books, 1993

England, Allison, *Aromatherapy for Mother and Baby*. London: Vermilion, 1993

Fenwick, Elizabeth, *Mother and Baby Care*. London: Dorling Kindersley, 1995

Gimbel, Theo, *The Book of Colour Healing*. London: Gaia Books, 1994

Goodrich, Janet, *Natural Vision Improvement*. Newton Abbot: David & Charles, 1987

Holdway, Ann, *Kinesiology*. Dorset: Element Books, 1995

Howard, Judy, *Bach Flower Remedies for Women*. Saffron Walden: C. W. Daniel Company, 1992

Illingworth, Ronald S., *The Normal Child*. London: Churchill Livingstone, 1987

Jackson, Lucy, *Childsplay*. London: Thorsons, 1993

Jackson, Lucy, *Medau*. London: Thorsons, 1992

Kaplan, Dr Robert-Michael, *Seeing Without Glasses*. Oregon: Beyond Words Publishing Inc., 1994

Kitzinger, Sheila, *The New Pregnancy and Childbirth*. London: Penguin, 1989

La Leche League, *The Art of Breastfeeding*. London: Angus & Robertson, 1988

Lee, Catherine, *The Growth and Development of Children*. London: Longman, 1984

Liedloff, Jean, *The Continuum Concept*. London: Penguin, 1986, and USA: Arkana, 1989

Machover, Ilana and Drake, Angela and Jonathan, *The Alexander Technique Birth Book*. London: Robinson Publishing, 1993

Mansfield, Peter, *The Bates Method*. London: Optima, 1992

McClure, Dr Nicola and Burton, Jane, *A Baby's Story*. New York: Simon and Schuster, 1989

McIntyre, Anne, *The Herbal for Mother and Child*. Dorset: Element Books, 1992

Newman Turner, Roger, *Naturopathic Medicine*. London: Thorsons, 1984

la Tourelle, Maggie, *Thorsons Introductory Guide to Kinesiology*. London: Thorsons, 1992

Wells, Henrietta, *Homoeopathy for Children*. Dorset: Element Books, 1993

Wills, Pauline, *Colour Therapy*. Dorset: Element Books, 1993

Index

Acknowledgements

EDDISON·SADD EDITIONS would like to thank the following models:

Kim Adams, Sharon and Molly Beardsmore, Lorraine Geard, Mark Gough, Daniel Heydecker, Asha Mamtora, Lala and Katie Manners, Keiran and William Osborne, Kathryn and Isabella Rai Whitehouse, Claudia Selby, Emma Smith, Joshua Somersall-Weekes, Kikelomo Thomas-Smith, Ethan West.

EDDISON·SADD EDITIONS

Project Editor............... Zoë Hughes
Copy-editor.................. Sue Moore
Proofreader.................. Sophie Bevan
Indexer...................... Dorothy Frame

Art Editor................... Pritty Ramjee
Mac Designer................. Brazzle Atkins
Photographer................. Laura Wickenden
Illustrator.................. Julie Carpenter
Production................... Hazel Kirkman, Charles James